PASTORAL CARE AND CONTEXT

Pastoral Care and Context

Otto Stange
(Editor)

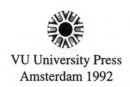

VU University Press
Amsterdam 1992

VU University Press is an imprint of:
VU Boekhandel/Uitgeverij bv
De Boelelaan 1105
1081 HV Amsterdam
The Netherlands

Tel. 020-6444355
Fax 020-6462719

Printed by Wöhrmann, Zutphen
Lay-out by Avo-text, Amstelveen

Isbn 90-5383-041-3
Nugi 636

Contents

By the way

You are examining a book on pastoral care.

It is not the first one ever to be published, and it will probably not be the last.

But developments in this field take place so rapidly that *not* taking notice of what is going on means rapid delay.

Once every four years members of the International Council on Pastoral Care and Counselling meet for a substantial international conference. In 1991 this conference took place in the Netherlands. The addresses, delivered by the main speakers, are collected in this book.

The - Dutch - basic paper deals with Pentateuch - characteristics as paradigm for pastoral care, adding a contribution in the field that is perhaps the least developed of all in this area: that of theological reflection. It is understandable that among workers whose major aim is action, there would be some resentment to tackle, not the widespread 'how to' questions, but the more remote issues of underlying prolegomena and consequences. Here is somebody who leads us into the field, inviting us to follow.

England - the other European contributor - works on the younger issues of women in relationship to traditions in pastoral care.
Here it becomes apparent that, in a continent which considered itself wealthy in traditions, and established, new issues may cause great changes.

In Clinical Pastoral Education - regarded as the main direction for the development of Pastoral Care for the International movement - North American categories, presumptions and methods have been standard up till now. As we read the contributions of the other continents, we become aware that circumstances (or: the context) are often so entirely different that great adaptations have to take place if anything should be accomplished at all.

India - the Asian participant - has to deal with complicated caste-systems that, although officially abandoned, still rule over a Hindu-dominated society. It takes great skill and sometimes diplomacy to provide pastoral care here, especially to those oppressed most: women and those of the lowest casts or even below that.

Africa has, of course, a long tribal tradition and a broad spectre of native religious forms, mostly older than imported Christianity. Pastoral care is just one of the options, mostly in competition with other providers.

In Chile - the South American contributor - the wounds of political outrage are still by far not healed. Pastoral care has to deal with people in circumstances which never appear in traditional literature.

Finally North America dwells on another Old-Testament question: Can we learn from the prophets. We can, considering attitude more than action.

All these essays were brought together in Holland, providing caleidoscopic and concentrated listening to all present. They took the abundance home with them, thus spreading it over the world. The spreading will continue with all those who start reading - and thus participating.

Welcome to some very interesting reading!

Otto Stange

Case Based Reflections on Contextual Pastoral Care: My Experience in Chile

Jorge Cardenas Brito

I acknowledge the invitation to contribute to this encounter. It has forced me to think, from a pastoral care perspective, about my work as a layman, and its context, during the last years. A layman in the process of receiving formal theological training.

I have used the opportunity to review briefly my 'pastoral care' activities, searching for implied models or some coherence in those options and actions, in relationship with the context, in an effort to discover the results of the contextual pressures, but always from the personal perspective and interpretation of the events, according to my experience of them.

These are provisional and very incipient thoughts, due to the multiple requests arising from the church, ecumenical companionship, church leaders, social actions-organizations and agencies, from patients, local congregation, students. Although, a minute for thinking about the whole work at so many levels is an unavoidable need. These are frequently the circumstances of pastoral agents in situations like the Chilean, circumstances I try to analyze. Circumstances of constant fight for survival.

For those reasons this is a predominantly discursive address, made underway, from memories, thoughts, and in the middle of various requests. I will write, not from theoretically elaborated relationships and context, but from perceived context and relations. I try to suggest, more than being analytical or systematic. Not because I am against analysis. I think it will be productive for the pastoral care in Latin America in the future, if reflection is given on what has been done in the moment of requirement, thus building guidelines systematically.

This can be discussed, but I believe we are in the initial stage of pastoral care adequate to its situation, for minority churches. Churches marginal to their societies in almost all the cases, but churches in constant growth.

It is a frequently heard critic, that the immediate demands of pastoral care inhibit the systematic development of the thinking about the practice, the elaboration of general principles and the building of the theoretical body that informs it.

I believe the incipient and suggestive thinking about the experience can be the basis for more ordained and specific developments à posteriori. Maybe they will be more independent from the first world developments, more expressive of the total reality and its complexities, able to integrate the developments of systematic theology and biblical reading in Latin America during the last decade. I see this stage as necessary to develop a creative practice of pastoral care and counselling, less repetitive and more connected to its situation. A situation that is now changing rapidly in Latin America.

With curiosity, while reading these reflections, I have seen how much of my own pastoral activities, thoughts and options have been guided by those developments, and by an effort to conciliate apparent antinomians and exclusions between individual and structural pastorals and between needs posed at different levels, but always starting in the situation perceived, more than from an ideological, theoretical or determined theological formal point of view.

I would say the same from bibliography. Sometimes I simply mention ideas belonging to others and which I find in the net of my pastoral actions and options, weaved in my thinking about that practice and the practice of others that are present to me. Without being able to say how much is mine, I am sure that most belongs to others, good or bad understood. Those whom I mention and whom I do not, will forgive me.

Describing the subject of the pastoral experience under examination

Something to have in mind about this address is that it is presented by a layman. Layman during the period of experience under test, and who in some way came out of the situation, transformed into pastor 'by right', to distinguish the formal and posterior condition of ordained pastor. Curious effect of the situation and the pastoral action on the pastoral agent, but very common and suitable for the circumstances of our churches.

Although paradoxical for pastoral care understood in a professional sense, but in agreement with one of the pastoral guidelines and the situational requirements of the churches in Latin America, this is the pastoral experience and pastoral thinking of a layman.

I am a physician, reflecting on his experience as a pastoral agent, but without formal theological education.

Thus it is, somehow, the pastoral experience of a physician working in different areas, and always in the perspective of a wide and extensive health conception. Due to necessary options imposed by the situation, and which interpellate him as a physician and as a Christian, interpellations that concern as a pastoral dimension and that assumes from the perspective of care, he is near the field of pastoral care.

In this case the word 'pastoral' is a difficult word, even though a positive reaction towards pastoral care by the lays can be observed. It would be cautious to discuss the convenience of the use of the word pastoral, and the change which somebody proposed, and to speak about a practical contextual theology of care, keeping 'pastoral' in reserve for the minister.

In any case, I have preferred to maintain the use of the word. I seek to define the actions of care performed on a given situation and context considered by a lay as 'pastoral'. Result of a Christian commitment to be assumed and exercised by the church, resulting from the situation.

Thus, pastoral dimensions of a Christian vocation somehow are expressed in concrete actions and determined criteria that we can call 'pastorals'. It is incumbent to all believers and their communities.

The concrete experience is given when trying to answer to a series of facts of the community's life of the church, of the people and of the Chilean society. Specifically when trying to respond to the needs perceived in these three areas.

In the contextuality perceived in the situation of the Latin American church I believe we are still in the stage of reflecting on the necessity of a professional justification of the pastoral. I do not have doubts about the need of a systematic and disciplined knowledge, as it is in science. We try to make these professional actions compatible with the universal priest-hood of believers. This seems a wider reality to us, and therefore the professional understanding seems to us subordinated to it and not the other way around.

The subordination of the ministry to the universal priesthood has been understood as a delegation of functions, which seems unsuitable to me because the vocation cannot be delegated. Generally the whole pastoral responsibility ends, being delegated, and not only some specific functions. This impression, that the pastoral of the laics should be subordinated to that of the minister, still remains when reading the description of pastoral care from the seculars in the most recent texts (with some exceptions, of course).

The pastoral function is a function of the people; in any case a wider function than a function of attendance or assistance within the pastoral task of the minister.

To make compatible the theory of the pastoral action with pastoral of the church as a whole, avoiding the clerical paradigm, is the task. Also to favour complementary actions of specialized ministries and the pastoral actions of the people of the church. That is our attempt, living in the midst of a tradition centred in the priest who is central in our countries.

In this situation the requirements and modalities of theological education originate from the practice and concrete necessities, given by the pastoral work of the church, and not from the perspective of training a professional. It seems to me that something of this reality is manifested in the experience lived.

Finally, this is a reflection on the situation that presents specific demands to the pastoral routine. Product of a Christian vocation which only progressively reaches the self-understanding of being pastoral. Therefore, it requires hierarchical rearrangements first. I believe that acting as lay from this perspective is different than acting out from other perspectives. It involves a series of differences in the way many issues are considered, for example leadership and church policy.

In these issues becomes involved according to his or her own perceptions, selections and actions, gradually developing a vision of what is pastorally necessary, self-understanding and insight.

The situation of the experience according to the perceived context

In the course of our reflection we now enter into the stage of description of the circumstances among different areas:

- The Chilean society and its political and economic situation.
- The reaction hereto of the non-Roman Catholic churches and their understanding of pastoral care and
- The situation of the people and of individuals.

In the first place, Chile has lived, between 1970 and 1990, through two periods marked by the attempt of introducing deep changes. One tried to establish the socio-economical and political life within a socialist conception, until 1973. The second, capitalist, from that year until 1990, and installed by an authoritarian military regime in a coup d'état, undid the first.

Nowadays, we live a process of transition towards a democratic adminis-tration, in an economy of free market, integrated to the international economy. It is said - and a fact - that in the big figures it has been successful and is now developing towards a social economy of free market. Questions remain about the ecological and human face of this success.

Both first stages were of great intensity concerning the changes carried out in the structural, the mobilized political forces or the repression exercised. They were accompanied by big repercussions on people's life, according to their options, and also in the lives of Christian communities. Many had no options at all.

The years of the so-called "Chilean way to socialism" were years of confrontation among political actors, and mobilization of some sections of the population. Great disarrangements in the economy were provoked by all the actors involved in the confrontation. Chilean society became extremely polarised, including the churches. Confrontation-style became common in all areas.

The years of the military regime were marked by another series of great changes in the economical and administrative structures of the country, and of a radically contrary sign to the former. And this in the frame of a strategy of a civil war, according to the conceptions of the doctrine of national security.

The imposition of the economic model was made at great social price, and with contained demands. Demands that were contained also during the process of economic readjustment due to the control of the military force. The evident correlation is that of large social inequalities, imposition of structures and ways of life, violations of human rights, cultural control and censorship, suspension of political activities, etc.

A climate of institutional, political, terroristic and criminal violence seems to have been unchaining, and maybe still is generating, a feeling of insecurity. In many areas this seems to lessen since the democratic restoration, but still the government has been urged to increase the police force in an effort to control delinquency.

Also many public health problems - related with the consumption of alcohol and drugs by youth groups - need to be addressed. In a sense they are part of the social damage of a successful development without a human face.

The pastoral answer of the evangelic churches

Different pastoral performances of evangelic churches correspond to this overall situation. We try to describe them in their general features, trying to identify the concepts of pastoral care, the strategies of action from the point of view of pastoral care.

I will distinguish groups according to their position within the established general situation, without differentiating among the evangelical churches on the basis of other criteria.

First period

During the process of changes that took place between 1970 and 1973, apparently there are no great conflicts, except discussions within the church by movements which originated from the sixties and which postulate new alignments for evangelic churches in the social context.

Second period

Nevertheless, the apparent tranquillity in the relationship churches-state is broken with the action of the military in 1973. For diverse reasons a group of leaders from protestant and pentecostal churches appear soon, representing the majority of the evangelical movement, who express approval and acknowledgement to the Chilean military process.

This so remarkable change, regarding the position maintained towards the socialist government, can have different explanations according to different points of view. I think that from a pastoral perspective, somehow the relationship with the former government must have been marked by expectant ambivalence.

If the statement made by some - those who say that the majority of popular evangelic movements represent people disenchanted with political processes and parties which could not give an answer to their contingent needs - is right, it is understandably an ambivalent reaction, regarding the expectancy frustrated again (if there was any sympathy for the process from 1970 to 1973).

First stage
From that moment on some leaders and/or ecclesiastical groups received space and public presence as never before by evangelical churches. Seen from the socio-religious perspective, these acts have been defined as suppletory of a religious legitimation denied by the traditional religious actors. A secondary legitimation lies in the response to the searched, and never gotten, acknowledgement by secondary religious actors, minority and marginals in the Chilean religious context. This in spite of being almost a 17% of the population.

However, this does not give an interpretation from a pastoral point of view. It does not proceed beyond a qualification - or disqualification - of the conduct itself.

From a pastoral perspective it is perhaps possible to define concepts of implicit pastoral care, strategies and priorized addressees of pastoral care, and clear options. These options can be tested for their adequacy to a broad perception of the context and to the Word. However, it is also right to understand them as concrete pastoral actions in a situation of crisis that reveals defined theological and pastoral criteria. This is of great importance in the coming consultations between different evangelical actors about very delicate issues in the perspective of reconciliation and unity.

Second stage

After the described initial stage of support follows one of silence of a large sector of the churches, parallel to the public action now limited to big events on the part of a remaining sector of the group constituted in the first stage. This happens because some groups, in silence and progressively, move away from the initial position, keeping an ambiguous attitude towards military authorities.

Somehow they were retaking their habitual position of social disregard, altered just transitorily by the necessities of the crisis and to assure a religious space free from control or restrictions; space so hardly conquered in the previous decades. Things had returned to their usual order. The often criticized social disregard had now greater justification in view of the circumstances. The world had revealed its condition in a dramatic way again. From here the pastoral criteria of these churches will arise.

Parallelwise, during the whole period para-ecclesiastic institutions under the protection of the churches have appeared with clear pastoral action, directed to the victims of the situation in the political field, but with a relation to the churches that must still be analyzed. These institutions assume from other instances the pastoral actions which the churches themselves seemed unable to assume, be it by an attitude of disregard and political resignation or because of a poor and discriminatory legal status of the protestant churches in Chile. In fact this status makes them very week towards the government.

Third stage

Almost ten years later, in 1985-86 approximately, a clear minor sector of the churches (in existence and cautiously active from the beginning, and with special relations with the para-ecclesiastical institutions) assumes a critic position towards the national situation in public, with a different pastoral strategy, issued from a different analysis of the situation and also from changes perceived in it.

An analysis is currently being made of its declarations, documents and the use of Scripture within those. Different phases can be discovered in the actions of this group: One of conquest of a manifest space and voice, another of intense effort to change the national and international public image of evangelical churches as 'The evangelical church which supports the military regime unconditionally'.

In its public expression, the will of this sector to assume a pastoral responsibility towards the society as a whole, of orientating pastorally the Chilean evangelical people for a concrete action in the socio-political context, in the tradition of respect to freedom of conscience of a Christian submitted only to Scripture, is evident.

An attitude, different from the traditional one, can be perceived in the activities and strategies, decidedly leaving behind the social disregard and in pursuit of independence from administrative authorities and political forces.

It assumes a clear public option against violence, in solidarity with its victims (in any sector). The key lines of this pastoral action comes to be peace, truth, reconciliation, freedom with justice, reparation to the victims and respect for human rights and nature. The difficulties to maintain such a position during a transitional process became evident in the last year.

The presence of this sector gains more relevance as the fixed date for the beginning of the formal processes of transition comes nearer. By means of a plebiscite and one election the people will give its opinion. That is the moment when the requirements from the different political actors, from the people in need of pastoral guidance, and also the attempts to influence the members and supporters of the evangelical churches are greater, and also greater the necessity to define pastoral guiding positions.

Third period

To the beginning of the transitional period, the requirements of (and towards) the churches change. Public spaces seem to narrow, activity becomes silent, contacts among different evangelical sectors are initiated in order to adapt to the new circumstances. The political actor - now government - cannot ignore the reality of the presence of the majority of evangelical sectors, independently of their previous attitudes. The necessary actor in the moment of the confrontation is now just one more in the religious reality of Chilean society.

The concrete individual pastoral actions

In this social and ecclesiastical context a decision had to be made. The initial need was to define the position of something to be called pastoral action. Of course, this understanding is in retrospective view. Simply stated, the need was to choose lines of action or to participate in one of the attitudes defined with respect to each stage in the church's response to the situation. It is clear to me that those decisions were made from a pastoral and also medical perspective, as I said at the beginning. The question was: what is pastorally adequate? It was not: what is theologically adequate? Of course I understand that behind the question and behind the answer there are specific theological assumptions, but those surely belong mainly to what we can consider practical theological thinking. But which are those ideas?

Once the decision was made for the third stage, the task was to answer to the needs arising from the situation, as seen from that new perspective. Needs at different levels, including assuming leadership, caring and counselling leaders, giving pastoral orientation to large and distant groups. The task became a challenge: to transfer experience, practices, techniques and knowledge of care at the individual level to the acting leadership, and pastoral care of large anonymous groups that could be reached only by public media, journalists, radio, etc. There was the need to interpret situations and events in individual counselling and orientation to leadership and pastoral guidance, and also to develop a way of confronting opposed groups pastorally.

All this while in the meantime still doing medical, and what we can consider traditional church work, and maintaining a sense of coherence in all what was being done and decided. Without getting confused in respect to the identity of the work that is being done, as pastoral work.

One of the greatest problems was to overcome the division between individual and structural. It is still difficult to see both correlated and as part of the same pastoral action. It was and is also difficult to avoid the confusion with political action. Although it was done at what can be regarded as a political level, it still remained pastoral as seen by the pastoral agent. I believe that clarity in mind about this is fundamental for the concrete action. The risk of confusion of the agent himself is constantly present. The question about the final identity of the actor as one doing pastoral care and counselling at that level, is not without consequences.

A question that arises constantly is the question of coherence, in an effort not only to see what is and was done as appropriate to the context, but also as a coherent personal action, and not as a diffusion of identity and vital project.

Reflective-meditative analysis

How can one, who has consciousness of having adopted the 'right position' pastorally, accept to be postponed by the necessities of a political transition? Here is where criteria of evaluation of the context, of the kind that is accepted in the pastoral practice enter clearly. Criteria which are not oriented by the usual strategies of management of power, but by a therapeutic concept of the management of the same, and of its termination. Now, the implications of a criterion of pastoral care applied to leadership are clear, and like this it can continue being a possibility of contextual pastoral care.

On the other hand: how to keep the pastoral action at the level of society focused on a defined theological criteria, as it was done in the years before (confrontation and denouncement), but in a new political context which seeks to generate consensus and not confrontation among groups of common interests, remaining at the same time independent from the new authorities and without being confrontational and functional other than to groups of the extremes?

It could be useful to observe that, during the whole process, churches never forget themselves as subjects and objects of the pastoral action. And this, although it seems inadequate, is in the right line because the evangelical churches in America Latina are not in a situation to 'make a preferential option for the poor'. They have never been the churches of the wealthy. They are marginal churches, socially and legally discriminated, they are poor themselves. (There are exceptions with some churches that can be identified with migration groups).

More than a problem of options, it is a question of identities which must be solved, to make the pastoral attitude clear. In this way I consider the 'division by options' within the evangelical movement as irrelevant, at least to be avoided considering our churches.

It may seem only a subtle change in the appreciation of the situation, however I think there is a great difference in the planning of pastoral actions and leadership as pastoral activity within the protestant ecclesiastical communities, when the identities change. "The therapeutic alliance is different", to speak in those terms.

Another pastoral line is given by the present situation for those marked by the psychosocial consequences of an authoritarian regime. The necessities of reconciliation, the service to the truth as a step for a genuine reconciliation and restoration, the search for justice and the construction of peace in the process of building a democratic society together, are specific pastoral needs to which pastoral agents and churches have to contribute from their specific field.

For example: what does it mean, theologically, to be somebody returned from exile? What meaning has faith in that experience? How is pastoral work to be done in that case, which are the pastoral orientations in this case? And again: this without obstructing the actions of other social agents, and considering the strong wish of large groups not to risk anything that can endanger the transition which was so hardly achieved by a past sorrow, or to evoke what they want to forget.

Here the present pastoral challenges begin. The strategies or implicit pastoral care positions must demonstrate - or not - their capacity to answer to needs posed by these circumstances. Needs that again embrace the churches, their members, their leadership, those who request repair, truth, justice, and the residual fear, fear of new injustices, or vengeances, of frustrated expectancies, etc.

Then, how to solve the opposition among lines of pastoral action? I bring in mind that when the pastoral actions of the different ecclesiastic protestant actors are considered all together, a certain logic appears in the sequence of assumed attitudes.

In fact, the first reaction, to take care of the religious space won in past decades and apparently threatened by an administration with enough legal instruments to be threatening, given the stunted legal position of the protestant churches, proves to be successful. A necessary basis for the action that will come later is strengthened.

Also the stage of silence seems adequate because it establishes an incipient process of separation, and stabilization of the protected space for some final prophetic action. It is clear that each action is done by different actors, all of them present from the beginning but acting at different moments. Thus, still given the simultaneous action of these actors, the one seems to give the previous step for the action of the other. The results are adequate to them and to the broader context, due to the clear identity of these churches as marginal. In all the cases they start from the position of the ones without power.

At least in this case the perceived context and the life context would be the key for the sequential actions, although each begins from different pastoral explicit schemes. The context is one of the keys because it is context of the same addressee and agent. There is coincidence of contexts.

Thus the context is not independent, but always a perceived context and it will vary according to addressee and agent. Therefore what is important is coincidence, and not that they are the same. Because of this multiple level, pastoral action will be more complete in a way that more pastoral agents have the possibility to respond to the perceived necessities, building together the coincidence of contexts.

This was what happened. There was a proliferation of agents, which should not be evaluated only as fragmentation. Maybe it is a need of contextual action. Then pastoral freedom will be a guarantee of plenitude or fullness, although there is always the chance of deviation or failure of responsibility. In some cases it is only a guarantee for a possibility. Then fragmentation like the one of the protestant movement in Chile can be seen, at least in some stages, not only as harmful.

The ecclesiastical situation corresponds, apart of what has been said during the description, to a reality of fast growing, fundamentally national churches. Churches born in the country and disconnected from the missions and for years outside ecumenic participation.

In a poor society and in sectors with a low level of organization, this quick growing group of statistically significant size makes pastoral requests unknown before. This provides also new opportunities for the group (Chile approx. 17%). The group reaches a social signification just because of numbers.

To have consciousness of the situation is in itself a necessity and it already establishes tasks and/or responsibilities. It determines demands at the level of capacity of the leadership and in the plans for its developments and practical capacity.

On the other side, this growth establishes big requirements of pastoral attention to individuals, families and groups. Attention to necessities which on a first phase are not perceived as connected to social problems, given the case of urgent action. This situation also presents formative needs of leadership.

The described situation suggests formative needs in the work of a department of practical theology. Where to concentrate the scarce formative time and resources assigned to pastoral care? At the individual or at the structural levels? Which are the strategies to reconcile alternatives? Can a contextual approach like the one used to search for coherence in the action of many pastoral agents provide them? A combination of graded contextual practices and a broad field of flexible alternatives and freedom to choose, and interdisciplinary classroom education could be the answer. To approach relevant topics of the context from an interdisciplinary methodology and with central pastoral care objectives can provide the contextual coincidence we need to avoid choosing between the individual and/or structural.

Another thing that appears from the analysis of our situation is that at a certain moment the pastoral alternatives were clear because the situation itself was modelled in terms of 'yes or no'. The main topics were precise and the possibilities of the church limited. The orientations were also clear.

Missing the central focus of the perceived context, in the field of pastoral care, around which the options and strategies were given, the arrangement of interests or points of pastoral action in the context change. They become oscillating, and time passes until a new field is organized around which options and strategy will be circled.

The constitutive focus or axis of the new pastoral action seems to be threefold: 1) challenges from the area of health, 2) the problem of the family (punctually the matter of divorce) and 3) freedom of religion (the legally discriminated existence of non-Roman Catholic churches). Especially this last focus is in continuity with that of former periods, and it seems to be narrowly connected with the possibilities of pastorals and future participation of protestant churches. Therefore it is understandable that around this focus of the global context, new concrete pastoral actions and coordinations among agents are given. The question is how to approach this new situation and how to gain action from a pastoral care perspective.

Another coincident observation with this concept of this field and of its oscillation and change, and therefore in the perceptions of urgencies of pastoral action, is apparently given in the change of the proposed themes for papers and essays of the students at the seminary. They have moved from Bible to practical theology, with a great diversion of themes. It is clear that this preliminary observation must be submitted to test and it must prove to be disconnected from other variables or circumstantial factors.

In a situation of change and transition the topics and questions diversify and compete among each other. This shall be common sense in normal circumstances but after 18 years of polarised alternatives they are seen in a new perspective. The necessities of new constructions and decisions regarding a great amount of material, ask for new criteria of priorization for the definition of areas of pastoral care action. In this situation the flexibility of the applied pastoral model is extremely important.

But, in general, what has happened on a large scale is repeated. The pastoral care directed to individuals and their necessities is seen as opposed to a pastoral compassion directed to the structural. The result is a rigid oscillation between one and the other exclusively.

Basically, there is a tendency to see the individual and the social or structural community as blocked divisions, they do not meet. The necessary distinction for understanding has ended in fragmentating the perception of the contextual reality. Then, in pastoral care, the choice is between mutually exclusive options. Who opts for working in with the individual has opted for excluding actions in the structural and vice-versa.

This is not contextual reality, not contextual pastoral care. Unfortunately I have seen many young pastors caught in this false alternative.

But the division seems to go further on. There is a tendency to see as separate actions the structural communitary ones, and those communitary actions which focus on the group or its members. I think the problem is not resolved by making more distinctions by describing psychological, religious and structural levels to be covered by the pastoral care of the churches, because by this polarization distinctions in the context, which end by being exclusive, are still being introduced. The inverse movement is required. The inverse movement consists of looking for ways of rebuilding the totality from the fragmentation of the analysis. I believe that this can be done by regarding the complete context as the field of pastoral care, and by a multidisciplinary approach and investigation of this context, in order to widen the view and to find more, pluralistic, alternatives.

Some final considerations

At least three elements are involved with the present pastoral situation:

- The massive growth and the great need of pastoral care by church-members in severe poverty.
- The marginal position of these churches, being a minority.
- Marginality and poverty are shared with large groups in society. Action has to originate from there.

Besides, religious pluralism and beginning secularisation are so recent that we haven't yet started considering them and their impact on pastoral care. What does it mean that pastoral care is given in a context of generations' suffering? Will it provide a sense of meaning and identity, without fostering conformism?

I believe that in given circumstances pastoral care needs the opportunity of several different options; that there is not 'only one specific pastoral orientation'.

1. Prophetic word and pastoral care action

In the present circumstances, the prophetic word needs to become pastoral in a different way. This is necessary if we want, as churches and as pastoral actors in the field of care, become agents of reconciliation. We have to work so that negation is avoided. Suffering and frustration should not be used with instrumental purposes, pain needs not to develop into exhibitionism. Prophecy is needed, but in a different voice.

The sufferings and the pain that first had to be denounced, are now in need of becoming intimate. Consolation becomes relevant, and the discovering of meaning fundamental. These actions, previously considered pastoral for crisis, have now to be seen in their transformational possibilities. They have to be seen as possibilities to generate changes, not as a 'calm down' pastoral care.

Prophecy must regain its meaning as a pastoral care-activity. This perspective should be aligned with the prophetic vocation. Only in this way the reductive understanding, already mentioned, will be overcome.

Polarization has occurred between prophetic denunciation and pastoral care action, although in my experience, as it was outlined, both were present in specific pastoral actions. Pastoral care has been too frequently identified with something related to the taking care of a certain type of childish members of the church, to be applied only to the church, and oriented to foster the participation, maintenance and attendance of worship. The 'prophet' appears as opposed to 'the pastor'. My experience reveals this to be false.

Pastors need to become free of those false confrontational alternatives, in order to build an integral concept of their task in our context. My perception of it is global and my pastoral answer in its specific options should remain also global, although it becomes focused. Fields are formed and in them I will find the places for my concrete actions of care. They will have meaning as consolation and as prophecy, if I take both seriously in the moment of deciding about the circumstances. In this case if I decide not to be prophetic when it is needed I cannot say I am pastoral, and vice versa.

The pastoral agent must feel and see that his particular and individual ministry is inserted in the context of the global ministry of the Christian community, but not in the sense of an adding of partial actions, but as an organic and integral answer to the context. He/she shall see his action as one of transformation of reality and of the global situation. She/he shall understand that many people, inside as well as outside their own circles and the church, do pastoral work on different levels and in different areas.

Individual pastoral initiative and group initiative must become meaningful within structured action. This can only be done with a broader perspective of the context, and this requires, in the case of trained pastors, field education in transcultural circumstances and in ecumenical space inside and outside confessional lines.

2. Some final remarks

Through the enlargement of the context, it was possible to find relation and coherence between a series of seemingly dispersed pastoral actions. Now I can answer the question that arises, when speaking of the context of pastoral care activities: Which is the text? If the pastoral act is an act of a caring relationship; it is that towards a certain reality surrounding the pastoral agent. Now context has become text of pastoral action. Text to be read at different levels and with many methodologies, some more appropriate than others, reading that will facilitate the pastoral definition of context. There will be a meta-text in which future and past become active in all the levels (individual and structural) and relevant therefore for pastoral care.

The enlargement of the context will always allow a better understanding of the concrete actions in our own pastoral activity. I presume that this way of looking at our own and others pastoral work can help to attain criteria, different from the confrontational ones without evaluation.

My own pastoral activities now appear to me as marked by the search to conciliate opposites; different levels, and needs in each of them. One complex text and many contexts, points of departure of different pastoral care initiatives. Only the enlargement of the context, to include more text, allows me to know them as acts with unity and not pure dispersion in a situation of social crisis.

Also, within actions of different type and nature, there is a special pastoral intentionality, in obedience to the Word and an internal sense of vocation.

Also, it becomes evident that in responding and acting, the resources, means and guiding lines of this intentionality I call 'pastoral', were concepts and intentions to foment, protect, prevent, heal and recuperate. This surprises me because they arise strictly from my medical under-standing. Then, the starting context provides a basis to respond to the pastoral intention?

I can see how, from the other side, this intention and beginning of understanding is ethically oriented, using resources to be found in the church and its tradition, and qualified by perspectives of hope, wholeness, justice, fullness of sense for individuals and their society, arising in their broad scope from theological disciplines, predominantly practical theology.

I hope, not to have given models, but at least to have shared my particular experience in a way that can help to understand how pastoral work is done, and seen, at least by one actor in the Southern part of America.

Thank you very much for your time and patience.

Contextuality: A Theological Paradigm

Maarten den Dulk

Ever since taking part in Clinical Pastoral Training, I have become deeply convinced that *communication,* as we came to understand it during the training, is the heart or, as we read in the Proverbs, the issue of life. Out of this issue of life are the exits to a world-wide scattered community of men which is divided amongst itself. For the sake of unity among this community the heart should be kept with all diligence. No communio without communicatio.

I say this in the *context* of Dutch society, seized with what Simon Schama calls: the embarrassment of riches, as reflected in imposing 17th century Dutch paintings. And in this frame of mind I experience communication as a fascinating myth - a mutual delusion in which it is natural to conceal contrasts rather than show them. The liberating sources are not tapped, but stopped up. There is no real communication if we do not appreciate this constriction.

Indeed, the C.P.T. in which I took part, does not deny the necessity for the pastor to become aware of his place and function in his particular context. In the Dutch tradition of Berger, Faber and Zijlstra the pastor is emphatically reminded of the universal cultural context in which pastoral counselling functions.

But this concept of the universal, cultural context is found to be too broad and too indiscriminate to find our bearings. Our appreciation of culture evaporates in the heat of pastoral counselling.

What counts is the person opposite me and his cause. I focus on his relations in life and his life's work. The present stage of his journey through life concerns me. His experience of life is my point of orientation. In fact, I exchange the concept of world-wide contextuality for a form of immediate contextuality. I conduct the conversation cautiously within the boundaries of the immediate situation of that particular meeting. And each different conversation will present us with a different situation. Indeed, this is how my verbatim accounts were dealt with during the training. The validity of my reactions as a pastor was measured against the unique situation of each conversation. All attention was focused on the communicative moment of that single meeting. The relation with the universal context of culture and society was certainly not denied. At times it was noted. But there was no follow-up in the orientation.

This is where we find ourselves beginning to criticize the CPT - as indeed we should be doing. Neither the concept of the universal nor the concept of the immediate, radical contextuality takes seriously the social, eco-nomic, historic and ideological definition of the situation where people meet, nor does it take into account the indelible mark that brands the lives of these people. If the CPT does not wish to remain blind to this reality, it will have no choice but to accept the model of contextuality as liberation theology has come to understand it. It is true that an inner affinity to liberation theology is felt in the CPT. One realizes that this path cannot and should not be rejected. And yet, here too, we find a border. If I use this one model as the decisive orientation on the reality of all areas in life, I shall be forcing my conversation partner, under any circumstances, to play a home match under the conditions set by this model. And somehow that is not right. The other one's face is becoming obscure. He may be drawing my attention to an area in life that has become invisible in my concept.

Already in this first superficial exploration of the notion of contextuality in the CPT there is the danger of getting lost. In each concept there will always be this 'something' I want to hold on to. This goes for the universal cultural as well as for the immediate radical contextuality. It certainly goes for the critical concept of liberation theology. But how to hold on to 'something' of these notions, as long as the different concepts seem to crowd each other out, or even exclude each other? How does it get me any further? What help does theology offer me here?

During the last few decades, we have become used in Holland to the cyclical reading of the five books of Moses. They offer guidance and help me to find my bearings.

I should make it clear that I try to understand the Torah, the Law, in its existential meaning, as St. James indicates: as the Law of Liberty! (James 1 : 25).

It now appears that this one Law of liberty unfolds in a multiplicity of stories. The glorious white light of the Law of liberty is broken up into different colours in the prism of the Pentateuch. The same community and the same world appears again and again in a different light. Following these colours, I am given some guidance during my quest. I find that the books of Moses offer themselves as a paradigm for what I should like to call: *differentiated contextuality.*

The Torah as paradigm for differentiated contextuality

I should first of all like to indicate briefly what I mean by this vision of the Torah.

In *Genesis* man comes to light as a living being, conceived and born within the context of social nuclear relations, within the network of intergenerational connections. In *Exodus,* on the other hand, the same man is seen in the sphere of labour, in the context of labour relations that are dictated by economic structures.

This differentiation within the story of the Torah enables us to make a distinction between - as could be said with some naivety - a communal world and a system-dictated world. Paying attention to the one cannot push aside the attention given to the other. Energy is made free to pay attention to the sphere of *life* and to the sphere of *work* separately, accepting the fact that the two areas are closely interrelated.

In the book of *Numbers* man and society become visible as people 'under way'. We see a generation who for some forty years make history, break up camp, go on their way, organised in social relationships, who settle down only to break up again - stretching out to the future. We learn about the context of the community 'under way' in their process of building up and change.

In *Deuteronomy* society becomes involved in the process of continuous 'learning'. In order to go on their way and continue there each generation must obtain and deal with vital knowledge. Here becomes clear the meaning of the community's learning process.

On the one hand this differentiation will enable us to pay separate attention to the dynamics of social organisation and renewal as a historical process, and, on the other, to the organisations of the cultural and rational learning process. Here we learn to appreciate the dynamic of the *Spirit*, there the clarifying function of the *Word*. There is no need to play off the one against the other. A meaningful distinction can be made within their mutual and unbreakable relationship.

Thus humankind in the Torah comes to light in the land of the four streams: men according to their natural and material aspect in their vital and system-controlled world: and men according to their historical and spiritual aspect in their process of learning and change. Man roams the world during his lifespan and gains different experiences in the field of *life* and *work*, of the *Spirit* and the *Word*. The land of the four streams, however, has its source there where the community of those people is refreshed by the stream of *communication*. Each of the four areas in life is drenched in that continuous, vitalizing refreshing stream. In each area the issue is communication. In each area that stream is different, but they stem from the same source. The heart of the Torah is communication - this is how we should appreciate Leviticus - and out of this heart are the issues of the multilateral contextuality of existence.

The story of the Torah is told in such a way that it enables us to perceive the various contexts of human existence separately. And so this narration separates itself from the myth, the true nature of which is found in the confusion of the various areas of life, a confusion which to us is irritating and odd. The Torah frees the way to a modern functional awareness of life. At the same time this narration fights against contemporary ideological efforts to encompass all reality within one and the same interpretation scheme. If we read the Torah in this way, it will offer itself as a paradigm for differentiated contextuality.

The Torah as a paradigm for Pastoral Care.

How can these five books of Moses show us the way in our pastoral care? Let me try to speak "five words with my understanding" (1 Cor. 14 : 19).

Genesis - life

The first word is Genesis: that is life within the network of the generations. I have come to understand Genesis as the record of man being entitled to beget sons and daughters. This book sings of man who as daughter and woman or as son and man is entitled to live generatively, as a free, responsible, and above all creative subject. Man is supposed to explore a future for a new generation of sons and daughters. If this entitlement is perverted, this same man acts in an unexpected and destructive manner, indeed, he perverts the relation between the sexes and the generations. In many ways Genesis tells us how that man and that woman live in a continuous dialogue and negotiation and battle with respect to intergenerational relations.

I must add that it was only through the contextual therapy of Nagy that it came clear to me how decisive *this* context is for my existence. Confronted with the genogram of my family and with the specific questions of the pastor as guidelines, I became really aware of how I fill page after page in the ledger of my existence, together with my brothers and sisters, parents and children. I felt the heavy pressure of mutual expectations and obligations, of deficits and credits, and the challenge this meant to my own responsibility. Since Nagy discovered for me the meaning of this context, I read Genesis with renewed interest as the ledger of the Torah.

In Genesis I am taught something specific about this context. In all kinds of variations the story teaches that this context of the nuclear relations is no neutral area, neither is it an objective and normative order of being, and it is certainly not an ambivalent ground of being. It is the place where the God of Israel meets people in the roots of their existence, as inevitable as the facts of life and death. It is the place where man learns to understand himself as the image of this God, and man represents God through this amazing entitlement to live a generative and creative life, to receive the past as the heritage of the previous generation, and to explore the future for the next.

In this entitlement given to me, I meet God, his creative act, his generative willingness, his loyalty through the generations, his justice, his future of peace. In this inevitable meeting with God I come to know the notions of loyalty and justice as the fundamental categories of my existence, here and now, in the network of nuclear relations.

The pastor who helps me to develop an ever increasingly sharp and clear perception of nuclear relations shows me the way to God the Creator. I cannot meet God outside this context, and within this context I can only understand myself as man destined for the image and likeness of this creative and loyal God.

Exodus - work

The second word, Exodus, takes me into a different context, that of work, where the employment contract dictates human relationships. Here I shall expect to find man as being entitled to work. His employment is part of an organisation. There is social commitment as well as an obligation to work efficiently: to live and acquire a place and a name under the sun, and in so doing make the world into a permanent human abode.

But as soon as man appears in this story, work turns out to have been thoroughly and totally disturbed. Tyrants - "a pharaoh who knew not Joseph" - have reduced the stranger in their midst to a labourer in *their* service, have taken away from him the free control he exercised over his own work, and forced him to accept a unilateral labour contract. In short, he is there to serve their interests.

The communal world of Genesis is being infiltrated and colonized by the system-dictated world of economic and administrative complexes. Man's entitlement to work together and for each other in social engagement is perverted into oppressive and inhuman service. The victims cannot but rise in revolt as a way to freedom.

The decisive meaning of this context is understood in the praxis of liberation movements, where we cannot do without the guiding role of Marx.

If there is mention of contextual theology, *this* context is referred to first of all. In the light of this discovery Exodus is read and appreciated as the fantastic story of successful liberation. It is encouraging. Throughout, Exodus concentrates our attention on the context of the labour situation, and its narrative strategy unfolds as follows:

- first we are told of the liberation from the inhuman working conditions in the house of bondage;
- next we hear the declaration of human rights on the mountain of God;
- and finally we are activitated to build the house where God and his people can meet; that fine work of craftsmanship as example of honest labour, which in the final instance should lead to Eucumene.

In that final moment the story has its greatest force. In the context of the labour situation, beyond the suppressive system and the laws of economy, man meets God. God as liberator, God, who himself works, liberating,

God powerful and God the servant, who makes the world into a house where people can live. God who himself has the plan for the house of meeting and involves his people. Human labour will be allowed to be, indeed ought to be, a creative reflection of the work of this God, of his liberating praxis. This intended symphony of God's labour and the labour of man forms the most intimate secret of Exodus. Wherever and whenever this secret is forgotten, society digs its own grave. Those, however who keep this secret, understand themselves in the context of their own labour situation as co-workers of God.

The pastor who becomes aware of his own position in this context, will help me, in my personal situation and in my work, to distinguish between collaborating within the oppressive system and collaborating with God. Only if I am fully aware of this context, can I meet God as Liberator and can I get to know myself as a free human being entitled to be God's co-worker.

Numbers - Spirit

I now turn to the last two books, Numbers and Deuteronomy, which deal with the spiritual aspect of human existence. The book of Numbers tells us what happens when the Spirit moves human society. We hear the long awaited call to go out to the promised land. But this cannot be set in motion just like that. It pre-supposes the organisation and mobilisation of the whole community. A community cannot be moved without the setting up of intermediate structures. Thus organised, they are on their way to the future, aware of the risks of such an undertaking. It cannot be done in one go, but it will have to be done in stages, in a continuous process of breaking up and leaving to go on again, wherever and whenever the Spirit so moves them. The book of Numbers takes us into the context of the process of building up and the process of change in society.

It was Martin Buber who established the connection between this context in the book of Numbers and our own context - and he did this both in his exegetic and his political and philosophical writings. His interpretation of the dynamics of the processes in society points us not to a neutral, faceless destiny, or to a predictable result of human planning, but shows us the force of God's spirit. This Spirit liberates people to go on their way: it is a binding force in the community. That Spirit chooses the path of history where we are surprised by unexpected turnings and vistas. On his long and unpredictable road it is not theories and systems but people to whom it has been given to understand the signs of the times and to share this understanding with the community. People who observe the working of the Spirit and who dare take the path to Utopia, as prophets do. Buber has shown me an interpretation of the book of Numbers as a journal of God's-people-under-way.

The unique and shocking fact in Numbers is that the way of the people is completely blocked by external resistance and inner conflicts. The dynamism of the Spirit directs its destructive force against the community so that practically a whole desert generation dies underway, not excluding Moses, Miriam and Aaron. The community does not reach its destination, but is annihilated in a vast crisis. To be sure, the book of Numbers tells us about a new generation who are mobilised to enter the promised land. But here there is no room for relativism. The old generation does die in the desert and there is no passage through the vast and radical crisis. A new generation must come into existence. Chr. Barth recognises in this antithesis New Testament statements about the impossibility of inheriting the Kingdom of God unless this radical change takes place.

The Book of Numbers tells of the history of Israel in the light of a great eschatological change. On their way to the future, in their decisions and hesitations, their cowardice and recklessness, man and society in this oppressive story are confronted with God's Spirit, inspiringly dynamic and consuming as fire. *In* the dynamics of the processes of building up and change of the community man becomes involved in God and his Spirit. In that history people meet God as their final judge.

The pastor who understands this context, has the guts to see, as if he were a prophet, the great crisis at the bottom of our personal history. This pastor will help me in my own biography to meet God as Spirit, in the secret, the cloud and in the destructive force of the fire. Here I become

conscious of history as the field where our decisions are taken that lead
to peace on earth or to the downfall of society. Here I shall need the pastor
who is aware of the deadly serious character of the crisis, and who does
not run away.

Deuteronomy - Word

Deuteronomy demonstrates that it is only through the Word that the
community becomes aware of her journey in the world. Moses is seen as
teacher, narrator, preacher - in the praxis of preaching the Word; and the
community is summoned to keep these words, to deal with them and to
pass them on. During this journey the community is not driven along by
a dumb and inarticulate spirit, but is addressed personally, in a human
and rational language, and is made aware of its responsibility. Through
the medium of the clarifying word man acquires wisdom. In this process
of "lernen" we become mature. Deuteronomy takes us into the context
of the learning process. It takes us into the house of learning.

This book does not precede the Torah. It does not function as the
Prolegomena, but as the Postil to the Pentateuch. In this 'lernen' the
precious experience that Israel acquires on its journey, is kept, given
structure and made fertile for the future.

It has been the rabbinical tradition that through the ages has exempli-
fied this 'lernen' which is nurtured by praxis; and here, therefore, we find
a different notion of 'learning' as it has been called ever since Aristotle.

Deuteronomy, read and understood as a manual, makes us familiar with
the reality of the Word. The word addressed to me personally will never
be neutral or 'objective'. It has a definite working. The word has a positive
and forceful working as a blessing, which brings forth life, which makes
the earth bear fruit and which opens up the road to the future. But the
same word may also have a negative force, and become a curse, which
blockades our way through life, the earth shall be iron, and death will
reign as enemy. With such words we are concerned in conversation,
argument, political speech, meeting, literature, and in the field of

education. Indeed, in one form or the other we seek to compromise, to escape this choice between words as a blessing and words as a curse. But Deuteronomy makes us aware of the uncompromising, original, glorious and awesome reality of the words whenever people meet. Israel - as the manual tells us - is confronted by the original reality of the word, the word in its primal power and revolutionary working. Israel is confronted by God who speaks to man. God who blesses and curses the annihilating forces. In that hour the Mosaic house of learning is founded. People receive the gift of the word, the gift to deal with the word as teacher and pupil in a lifelong process.

Through this gift we are closely connected with this primal reality in the daily usage of words. Consciously or unconsciously what we say is a continuous dialogue with what God says, his Word, his blessing and curse. That is the most uncomfortable and the most challenging lesson of Deuteronomy.

The pastor who is aware of this will not run away from his role as a teacher. In this context the pastor is explicitly teacher, catechist, preacher of God's word. He need not be ashamed of the profile that Thurneysen drew. I am only helped by pastoral counselling if the pastor makes me aware of the fact that God is very "nigh unto me, in my mouth and in my heart" (Deut. 30, 14).

Thus these four books of Moses can be understood as a paradigm for pastoral care.

We feel that here there is a challenge for the training in pastoral counselling. The pastor will have to learn and develop a sensitivity towards the multilateral character of the context in which people find themselves. He should be able to discern the fruitless conflicts between the various areas of life. He should also appreciate the danger of one of these areas being made absolute. It is a challenge which will have to be met.

Leviticus - communication

Now we have seen that the four streams which are the fertilizing force in the various areas in life stem from one and the same source. That is the source of *communication*. In life and work *communication* is the issue in word and in spirit. If pastors can come to this central source, they will have come closest to the typical quality of their work. Here we can no longer avoid pressing questions. How do pastors arrive at this central source. Who empowers pastors to discover this source and to pass on its renewing force? How will pastors be able to realize change, resistance and liberation at all? Are they themselves not caught up in the concealing and oppressing mechanisms of their own context?

Once again I turn to the Torah to find its centre, its source guarded by the impenetrable book Leviticus, the "priests codex", as it is sometimes called. If this should be taken as a hint for the pastors to clericalize their own profession, I refuse to take it. I cannot and will not understand this reading of Leviticus. I hear something different. Here, in the centre of the Torah, it is not a secret of the *priests* and their ability to communicate which is guarded, but here the secret of *God* is kept. Unapproachable in the centre: His presence, His Name, His Spirit, His Word! We cannot approach here. Here, if anywhere, we become painfully conscious of the embarrassment in the pastoral meeting; the embarrassment namely of finding ourselves powerless in the decisive moment to do what should be done, of realizing that methods, tricks or good advice are of no avail, when we must finally acknowledge that all clerical, professional pastoral care has been knocked right out of our hands.

When I am overcome by this paralysing powerlessness, this impenetrable book Leviticus begins to open itself for me. In the centre of this story a man comes to light. A man as image and likeness of God. At a rare moment in time, on the Day of Atonement, one man approaches the unapproachable secret of the name. It is no more than an image and likeness of God. But I try to envisage this image:

The man who here comes to the force is alone, carries his life's blood and that of the community, and with it approaches the place where God wants to meet man. We follow his approach toward the mystery of the most holy place.There something unusual takes place. The man sprinkles the place of meeting with a drop of his life's blood, from his own finger. Without touching that place. It is a shy and at the same time decisive gesture, and it is repeated seven times. He seeks to approach God as closely as possible, while at the same time keeping the required distance. The spark of life jumps across between the finger of that man and God's - in a way like Michelangelo painted the story of the creation. What Leviticus chapter 16 tells us here is a living metaphor of communicative action.

But on that same day and in that same place something entirely different happens. The man leaves this intimate and most holy place, takes his place in the centre of this community, between two animals, two goats. And everybody who is engaged in this event, sees how the destiny of the whole community and of himself is shown in the destiny of these two goats. They are separated and set apart - as in a painful bibliodrama - the one to approach to God, the other to vanish into no man's land, as scapegoat into the wilderness.

Everybody is invited to recognise himself in the one as well as in the other creature: himself completely in the figure of the new creature, the new man who approaches God and inherits the future of Gods's Kingdom, and again to recognise himself completely in the figure of the old crea-ture, the old Adam, who makes himself intolerable and who has no future. He who so understands himself in this dual destiny is torn by despair. This one man however, who is vigilant and who has taken his place between the two animals, radiates trust that in this crisis a wholesome change may take place from the old to the new and real life.

And so what happens here, in this form, is likewise a living metaphor of communicative action.

Here the outstanding feature is that both actions take place on that one day: man acts in atonement with intimate gestures; and man, clearly discerning, reveals the crisis in the community; by doing both, atoning and critical, this man arrives at real communication.

This is not within our power - as the epistle to the Hebrews says about Leviticus - but we have someone who can. We have someone who has identified himself with that solitary human being in the heart of the Torah who is anointed and therefore entitled to act in true communication.

What can be said of this ability, about the power of this anointed one?

Here the Epistle to the Hebrews (4:15 - 5:10) discovers the most intimate secret of Leviticus. It takes us to the source of life. It is the ability, it says, to be touched with the feeling of the infirmities of others, to empathise when the other person is powerless, lost, estranged from himself.

That is not the ability which is given to us as something extra by virtue of our profession or office; it is not something extra, it is less.

It is the ability to know what it is to be surrounded by weakness, to suffer, to pray and to plead one's case in tears, with death staring you in the face. This is how the anointed one acts. And in this way he has fulfilled the Torah. And so the heart of the Torah is opened as the source of true communication. And in His Name we are entitled to draw from this source of communication.

The Relevance of The Biblical Prophets for Pastoral Counselling

Edwin H. Friedman

I want to begin by saying what an honour I feel this is to be invited and to come to people from all over the world. I realize that there are all kinds of complications here of different nations and different cultures and different backgrounds and different languages and I will do my best to speak distinctly for those of you who do not find English that easy. So I must tell you if you do not always understand me, it may not be your fault. People who understand English very well often say they did not understand me. What I want to do in this lecture can be outlined very easily; I'm going to talk about something that I don't think anyone has talked about: the relevance of the biblical prophets for pastoral counselling. And then I am going to apply those ideas to working with people in a counselling situation and family therapy, and then I am going to apply the ideas that I developed in relation to the prophets to the whole family of psychotherapy. That is: to the civilisation of psychotherapy and where pastoral counselling fits within that latter context.

But let me begin first with some ideas about the biblical prophets. I remember back in rabbinic school, that the students who were most interested in the prophets as compared to the Torah as well as other parts of Jewish tradition, never went into counselling. And I noticed that those who decided to specialize in counselling never made much of the prophets. And then I realized, over the years, that that was not just a Jewish tradition, because I learned in my training of non-Jewish pastoral counsellors, that the same thing was true. That rarely did pastoral counsellors make the most important - or even a significant - part of their own education, the biblical prophets. To make sure that it was not just an impression that somehow came out of my brain, I went to the library of a major theological seminary in the United States, The Wesley Methodist Seminary in Washington, and I went to the card catalogue and looked, and there were threehundred cards under pastoral counselling. Not one of them mentioned the biblical prophets. Then I reversed it and I looked under biblical prophets, and there were twohundred cards and not one of them mentioned pastoral counselling.

I then went to look at the periodical literature and they had a man there who was a specialist in putting in the right software, as you may have seen you can do today for literary research, and he plugged in the term pastoral counselling and other similar terms and he plugged in prophets, biblical prophets. There were seven thousand references to the biblical prophets. That is seven thousand different articles. And there were four thousand on pastoral counselling. He then pushed the magic button which cross-reference then, and we came out with twenty one, O.K.? Out of eleven thousand articles there were twenty one! Vingt et un. Einundzwanzig. Twentyone articles out of a total of eleven thousand possible, that contained, in the title, both biblical (Old-testament) prophets or any such men and pastoral counselling. Now you could say: maybe somewhere in one of those books they did touch on the subject. Still eleven thousand titles and twenty one of them contained the two ideas together. I think I began to understand why these two areas of our life, of our traditions, are generally not put together. Because the prophetic was understood to be confrontation. That is, if you put the priestly on one side and the prophetic on the other, the priestly is generally assumed to have to do with comfort and the prophetic with disturbing, with confrontation.

I'm suggesting to you that the significance of the biblical prophets for pastoral counselling is not in their message. It is in their functioning.

We all know that most of their message had to do with social justice. It had to do with purifying the temple cult of practices that were obnoxious with practices that we all aim. I'm suggesting to you that the real significance of the biblical prophets is the way they functioned within the family of Israël in those days. Now, being Jewish, I never tried to make interpretations of Christianity. But it is my guess that much of what I'm going to say about the biblical prophets was also true about the functioning of Jesus. I'm going to try to highlight four characteristics of their functioning, of the way they behaved, the way they aberrated, the way they dealt with others. And then after bringing these together I'm going to show their significance for working with parishioners, for working with people, with families, and then I'm going to apply it to the family of psychotherapy itself.

I assume you all know that the biblical prophets are traditionally divided into three groups: Those that prophesied before 586, before the destruction of the temple, before Nebuchadnesar, and their message is almost exclusively a message of social justice. Then there are other prophets, and the prophets of that period of course are Hosea and Amos and Micha, to mention three. The exilic prophets are primarily Jeremia and Ezechiël. And their message, while containing some issues of social justice, has more to do with the hope and the change of heart that is necessary for Israël to be redeemed. And then there are the postexilic prophets, primarily Deutero-Jesaja (Chapter 40 and on in the book of Jesaja), who started during the exilic period and who tried to carry on a new model for the religion of Israël. Now I'm not going to separate these three groups of prophets as they are normally done. I'm going to talk about all of them in terms of what they had in common. And that is, even though their message is different - depending on the context - they all operated in exactly the same way.

The first outstanding feature, I think, of the biblical prophets is: they struck a balance between being separate and remaining connective. They somehow were able to separate themselves out, they were able to differentiate themselves from the rest of the people, from the kingdom, from the government, from the priests and maybe from the other prophets. They were able to separate themselves out from the rest of their family. Yet, they did not cut themselves off. In other words: they somehow maintained what I call - and I learned the term from M. Bowen whom some of you have heard of - a differentiated position. They were able to be different, to be separate, but to stay connected. The point of that is: anybody can be different; the trick is to be different and remain in a relationship. That is always the problem.

Secondly, what shows up among the biblical prophets, all of them, is their clarity. They are clear. They defined themselves very clearly. They got their message across very succinctly, very sharply. They knew what they believed and they defined their position simply and clearly.

What I want to point out is: they were not organizers, none of them. You could say that Ezechiël was setting the basis for some sense of organisation, and maybe also Haggaï and Zacharia later, but generally speaking they understood their job as not to organize others, but to take a position, to make something clear. That is the second thing that is true about the biblical prophets. They were not organizers, they were - well, the Hebrew word nabib from which the word prophet comes, basically means to "bubble up", it basically means to utter, to set forth. The idea of predicting is a later notion that is associated with it. But the basic notion is, they were "mouthpieces", to use the English slang. They spoke out the message that they heard, and what they believed.

The third aspect of the biblical prophets that I wish to emphasize is their emotional stamina. They stayed on course.

To give two examples: Amos and Jeremia. There is that marvellous chapter VII in the book of Amos in which Amazia, the highpriest, comes to Amos and says: go prophesy - meaning, do your commentary - in an other city, go to Beth-El, because the land cannot bear your words. We cannot stand listening to what you are saying. And Amos instead of defending himself, instead of trying to explain himself, says simply: I am not a prophet, I am just a shepherd. God told me to do this. And instead of weakening his message he gets stronger. Jeremia goes through many trials of both an emotional and illegal type. He is thrown in a pit, he is put in a stockade. And if you look in the book of Jeremia every time people come to Jeremia and tell him to stop, not only does he not explain himself, he gets worse.

What would that be like? I'm always saying to people who are attacked: if you explain yourself and get defensive, you give the other one the battle. Even if you get a better argument, if you buy their battle ground.

So for example: A woman attorney in a law firm is making all kinds of suggestions, and afterwards the men attorneys come up to her and say: you know, you have good ideas, but you are getting a little pushy. And she says to me: they had never said that to a man, that he is getting pushy just because he comes up with a good idea.

I would then say to her: Well, the next time a man comes to you and says you are getting pushy you should say to him: If you cannot stand this, wait till I get aggressive.

That is the way Amos and Jeremia functioned. When people tried to throw them off course, they stayed right on course in the best way to do that, because the reason is significant: it is not possible to do the first two things without getting sabotized, it's impossible no matter what culture you are in. If you try to differentiate yourself, to be different, to be separate, don't get caught up in the anxiety of everybody. If you try to say things that are unpopular or against somebody, just to state your own position, then it is absolutely predictable that you will have to deal with the third thing, which is: people will try to sabotage you. That is as true in a church, as in a marriage, as in a country as in anything.

So, the third aspect of the biblical prophets functioning that I wish to emphasize was their emotional stamina, their capacity to stay on course. The fourth quality that I want to mention - I do not put this on the same level with the first three, but it is important - they had the capacity to be outrageous. They had the capacity to be absurd. Hosea marries a prostitute. Jeremia goes barefoot if not naked through the streets of Jerusalem and I think there are one or two other examples of the prophets being outrageous.

The importance of being outrageous or the capacity to be outrageous, absurd, paradoxical, is that it helps you with the other three.

All of this, these qualities: being able to be different or to set apart; clarity, clarity of belief; staying on course and being outrageous are, I believe, four qualities that also go into leadership. But it is a different kind of leadership than we normally think. It is no a cohesive type of leadership, it is not even leadership by example, it is leadership by a kind of presence.

I believe the effect of the prophets on Israël was the nature of their presence. A non-anxious articular presence that was full of integrity. How can these ideas be applied to the world of counselling, both individual counselling situations and the world of psychotherapy? I'm going to shift now and I ask you to just keep this what I mentioned so far in mind, I will come back to them.

As you may have heard, I have written a book of fables. I'm going to read to you one of the fables in the book. Some of you have heard some of this and I apologize for that. This is the first fable in the book and it is called *The Bridge*. I read it to you because I think it captures, it illustrates, what goes on in all counselling situations, in all helping situations, more than any other image I could come up with. The fable goes as follows:

> There was a man who had given much thought to what he wanted from life. He had experienced many moods and trials. He had experimented with different ways of living, and he had had his share of both success and failure.
> At last, he began to see clearly where he wanted to go, what he wanted to do with his life. Diligently, he searched for the right opportunity. Sometimes he came close, only to be pushed away. Often he applied all his strength and imagination, only to find the path hopeless blocked. And then at last it came. But the opportunity would not wait. It would be made available only for a short time. If it were seen that he was not committed, the opportunity would not come again.
> Eager to arrive, he started on his journey. With each step, he wanted to move faster; with each thought about his goal, his heart beat quicker; with each vision of what lay ahead, he found renewed

vigour. Strength, that had left him since his early youth, returned and desires, all kinds of desires, reawakened from their long-dormant positions.

Hurrying along, he came upon a bridge that crossed through the middle of a town. It had been built high above a river in order to protect it from the floods of spring.

He started across. Then he noticed someone coming from the opposite direction. As they moved closer, it seemed as though the other were coming to greet him. He could see clearly, however, that he did not know this other, who was dressed similarly except for something tied around his waist.

When they were within hailing distance, he could see that what the other had about his waist was a rope. It was wrapped around him many times and probably, if extended, would reach a length of 30 feet. The other began to uncurl the rope, and, just as they were coming close, the stranger said: "Pardon me, would you be so kind as to hold the end a moment?"

Surprised by this politely phrased but curious request, he agreed without a thought, reached out, and took it.

"Thank you", said the other, who then added, "two hands now, and remember, hold tight". Whereupon, the other jumped off the bridge.

Quickly, the free-falling body hurtled the distance of the rope's length, and from the bridge the man abruptly felt the pull. Instinctively, he held tight and was almost dragged over the side. He managed to brace himself against the edge, however, and after having caught his breath, looked down at the other dangling, close to oblivion.

"What are you trying to do?" he yelled.

"Just hold tight", said the other.

"This is ridiculous", the man thought and began trying to haul the other in. He could not get the leverage, however. It was as though the weight of the other person and the length of the rope had been carefully calculated in advance so that together they created a counterweight just beyond his strength to bring the other back to safety.

"Why did you do this?" the man called out.

"Remember", the other said, "if you let go, I will be lost".

"But I cannot pull you up", the man cried.

"I am your responsibility", said the other.

"Well, I did not ask for it", the man said.

"If you let go, I am lost", repeated the other.

He began to look around for help. But there was no one. How long would he have to wait? Why did this happen to befall him now, just as he was on the verge of true success? He examined the side, searching for a place to tie the rope. Some protrusion, perhaps, or maybe a hole in the boards. But the railing was unusually uniform in shape; there were no spaces between the boards. There was no way to get rid of this newfound burden, even temporarily.

"What do you want?" he asked the other hanging below.

"Just your help", the other answered.

"How can I help? I cannot pull you in, and there is no place to tie the rope so that I can go and find someone to help me help you".

"I know that. Just hang on, that will be enough. Tie the rope around your waist, it will be easier".

Fearing that his arms could not hold much longer, he tied the rope around his waist.

"Why did you do this?" he asked again. "Don't you see what you have done? What possible purpose could you have in mind?"

"Just remember", said the other, "my life is in your hands".

What should he do? "If I let go, all my life I will know that I let this other die. If I stay, I risk losing my momentum toward my own long-sought-after salvation. Either way this will haunt me forever". With ironic humour he thought to die himself, instantly, to jump off the bridge while still holding on.

"That would teach this fool". But he wanted to live and to live life fully. "What a choice I have to make; how shall I ever decide?"

As time went by, still no one came. The critical moment of decision was drawing near. To show his commitment to his own goals, he would have to continue on his journey now. It was already almost too late to arrive in time. But what a terrible choice to have to make.

A new thought occurred to him. While he could not pull this other up solely by his own efforts, if the other would shorten the rope from his end by curling it around his waist again and again, together they could do it. Actually, the other could do it by himself, so long as he, standing on the bridge, kept it still and steady.

"Now listen", he shouted down. "I think I know how to save you". And he explained his plan.

But the other was not interested.

"You mean you want help? But I told you I cannot pull you up myself, and I don't think I can hang on much longer either".

"You must try", the other shouted back in tears, "If you fail, I die".

The point of decision arrived. What should he do?

"My life or this other's?"

And then a new idea. A revelation. So new, in fact, it seemed heretical, so alien was it to his traditional way of thinking.

"I want you to listen carefully", he said, "because I mean what I am about to say. I will not accept the position of choice for your life, only for my own; the position of choice for your own life I hereby give back to you".

"What do you mean?" the other asked, afraid.

"I mean, simply, it's up to you. You decide which way this ends. I will become the counterweight. You do the pulling and bring yourself up. I will even tug a little from here".

He began unwinding the rope from around his waist and braced himself anew against the side.

"You cannot mean what you say", the other shrieked. "You would not be so selfish. I am your responsibility. What could be so important that you would let someone die? Do not do this to me".

He waited a moment. There was no change in the tension of the rope.

"I accept your choice", he said, at last, and freed his hands.

Now for me that story seems to capture the position of most people in the helping professions. At one medical school in the United States, where it is used in training residents in family medicine, I understand they use the phrase "row-burn" when they see one another stuck with some patient. Where does it come from, this thinking in my head, and how is it related to the prophets?

I must now tell you something about my own experience in the field.
I have spent 32 years in one community, Washington D.C. metropolitan area and I have watched a whole generation go by. This is a kind of longitudinal coordinate to my experience.

Children whose Bar Mitswah's I effectuated when I first came to Washington, today have children in college. During this period I have watched many different presidents of the United States elected and I have watched different administrations come in. Each vowing to fix what the previous one screwed up.

And I have watched one new theory of psychotherapy after another come along. The outstanding feature of my thirty-two years in the Washington area is the absence of change. I have watched a whole generation go by, a generation and a half, and I have seen small changes, but I have seen no significant change in the way people deal with one another and I have seen that most change recycles. And that has forced me to ask some basic questions.

In the Washington area, particularly the part of Washington I live in, if you have a synagogue or a church there, then you can expect that every member of your congregation is either in therapy or is a therapist.
What has struck me is that, while most of the therapy that these various people go to helps them cope with their lives, it does not change what is passed on to the next generation. That has been one of the really interesting, sad but interesting, facts of my perception in the Washington area.
While most psychotherapy can be effective in helping people cope with their lives, it does not seem to change what gets passed from one generation to the next, and the next generation has to work out the same problems all over again. In other words: there is not an evolutionary process occurring.

The same thing shows up with churches and synagogues. I am called in as a consultant to all kinds of institutions - and every religious denomination in the world has institutions - that are pills, and institutions that are plums. "Pill" is an English slang term for something that is not very changeable.

I have spoken with bishops and district supervisors and placement committees and the hierarchies of various religious denominations. To my knowledge no bishop, no placement director, no district supervisor has figured out a way of changing a pill into a plum. The pills stay that way for generations.

It is as hard to take a very successful church or synagogue and make it go bad, as it is difficult to take a terribly virulent church and make it go good. What is this multigenerational process that most forms of psychotherapy do not seem to touch?

What does it take to interfere with what is passed on from generation to generation? It is not enough just to make people feel better. It is not enough just to help people cope with their lives. Not if you are from a religious tradition. There are some similarities that I see everywhere.

What I gave you just so far was a longitudinal perspective, a perspective of thirty-two years. But in the last six years I have had a horizontal perspective, because the book I wrote, *Generation to generation*, has been very well read in the United States and I have been invited into almost every state in the United States in the last six years. So that in the last six years I have had the opportunity to make presentations to every religious denomination, every one in America. I have also had the opportunity to make presentations and to talk to people in education, in psychotherapy, in medicine, in law and four years ago I came over here to Mannheim, to Heidelberg and I spoke to army generals. There are certain factors that seem to show up that are the same, no matter what the institution is. So not only do religious denominations not differ from one another in the following, neither do the different disciplines, whatever it is: education, religion or politics or anything else.

The first thing that shows up is that in system after system, in organisation after organisation, in institution after institution it is the most dependent, the most recalcitrant, the most passive aggressive that are pulling the shafts. And that is true everywhere, even in the army.

At the end of the second day of a workshop, a three-star American general, that is the head of three panzerunits, stands up and says: You know, one of our problems is that the sergeants keep getting the new recrutes out of bed in the morning and we tell the sergeants that we make them very good soldiers in the field. And then he turns to his fellow-generals and he says: but from what Ed is saying here we are not gonna have any more luck changing the sergeants than they are changing the new recrutes. That this man has three stars on his shoulder! How much more authority do you want?

He commands more death than exploded in all of Worldwar-II. How much more power do you want? And he cannot change the recalcitrant sergeant. So the notion that the problem is power or authority is not true. That is not the problem. The problem has something to do with the way we understand the human phenomenon. What is needed, I believe, is a new model.

You see, the effects of the prophets on Israël was to change their view of reality. It changed their model. For the God of Israël, before Amos, was a triable God. The God of Israël before Amos was no different than any other God of any other people. But after Amos and after Jeremia and after Jesaja, the God of Israël was now the God of the world. They changed in two hundred years a whole way of thinking. As one of my biblical professors said: "What Amos was saying in the light of his time was tantamount; it was as though he was saying that God was going to commit suicide! Because the thought of a God punishing his own people was unheard of if the God needed that people. And what the prophet said was: God doesn't need you. Not only that, God is not chained to a geographical area, but He could as well go into Babylon.

So the prophets through the four things I said before - if that was true about them - changed the whole way of proceeding things. I think a new way is needed of proceeding emotional phenomena.

Today what happens is all consultants, all experts in change. Whether they are experts in family life, organisational life, religious life or whatever, they do the exact same thing. They come up with administrative, managerial or technical solutions. The problem with managerial, technical and administrative solutions is that they do not change emotional processes. And unless you can change emotional processes, each new generation will recycle what the previous generation did.

Let me give you an example of what I am talking about.
Every year I get letters about conferences and books. What of the following topics: I have listed them alphabetically. Every year I get notices that I can read about or go to conferences about the following:

Abortion, adoption, aging, anorexia, asthma.
Conflict resolution: communication, depression, grief.
Living with: preschool as latency, phobia schoolage, phobias, adolescences, learning, home, leaving home and learning disabilities.
Under marriage: blended family, single-parent problems, divorce, marital stress and intermarriage. Pain.
Under personality: schizophrenia, borderlines, obsessives and hysterics.
Under phobias: trains, plains, being alone and so on.
Psychosomatic illness: in the head, in the gut, in the skin.
Sexuality issues: impotence, premature ejaculation, frigidity, vaginism, homosexuality.
Under substance abuse: drugs, liquor, food, children.
Suicide Violence.
Now in addition to that I'm also told that I can approach any of those subjects from a different school. So there is a second count.
Under psychoanalysis there is pruriency.
Under family therapy: system, structural and strategic plus.

Eye therapy, massage therapy, play therapy, acupuncture and traditional acupuncture and there is more. Well, maybe one is specializing on someone of the family, such as wife, husband, father, mother, son.

For those of you who remember the higher criticism of the biblical texts this is "psychotherapies J, D, E and P". It gives you a deeper analysis of the problem, but it does not give you a better understanding of the whole. I have a most serious thing to say about all this. Not only is it absurd to believe that you could become an expert in any of this. The more you make your confidence in your professional capacity based on how much of this talking, knowledge, information you have got, the more you are doomed to feeling inadequate. Again: The more you make your confidence in your capacity to help people based on how much of this tale you put in your head, then the more doomed you are to feeling inadequate, and the great irony is that this has become a form of substance abuse. It plays the exact same role in the minds of the helping professions as taking a substance does in the people you are trying to help. Because: we get anxious and therefore we read more of this, but we developed the threshold very fast and then we have to go out and read more of this, so that publishers have become pushers.

I would also like to suggest to you that this is a form of idolatry and is the exact same kind of idolatry that the prophets were opposed to. Because it is the belief that some way or another you can, through something technical, change something that is part of the soul.

What is happening in the world of psychotherapy is: it has got all caught up in the anxiety of the world, and the anxiety of the world always keeps focusing on something.

Twenty years ago, when I was first beginning to do therapy, there was never a conference without a sex therapist. Sex therapy was the end of everything and if only everybody had good sex lives everything would go great. And that lasted about seven years. Since then the focus has shifted to anorexia and then abuse, and so on. And it will keep you thinking. And everybody in their anxiety keeps focusing on something else. We are focused on ozon holes for a while in society, and something else will come along and everybody will forget about the ozon holes. So that society keeps focusing on something which its anxiety will just get bound through.

If the world of pastoral counselling is to be influenced by the prophetic movements it must avoid to be caught up idolatrously in the way psychotherapy has dealt with the anxiety of society, which is just to take the latest symptom that everybody is worried about and try to figure out how to fix it.

It is possible to come up with new models. It is possible to come up with new ways of thinking about much of this. What has happened is: we no longer believe in the pantheon of Gods.

There is another fable in de fablebook. Oedipus and Faust get together to discuss what happened to their myths and Cassandra comes in and talks about how society keeps denying the obvious and that in every age there is still that denial. And she talks about how in her days everybody believed in the Gods and they believed in Aphrodite, Mars, Venus and so on, and that today the Gods have simply changed their name and now they are called genes and gender and background and so on. And everybody still puts their faith into the hands of forces they believe they cannot control. That is exactly not what the prophets were trying to say.

What has happened today? One of the things that Cassandra winds up saying is: and Zeus the powerful king of the Gods today is called "a dysfunctional family of art". In other words, we still must have some force out there that we can attribute our faith to. I think it is Euripides who says: We are constantly moulding our character and calling it faith. That is twenty five hundred years ago.

What would be a different model? A different model is a model that focuses on trying to find the prophetic element in any family. Family therapy is not just a new technique, it is a new way of conceptualizing emotional phenomena.

For example: Here is an earthly family. This family is from the planet earth and the culture does not matter. There are parents, one or two, and children. In every family on this planet the following is true: Symptoms can show in one of three locations and only one of three locations. In a marriage in the health of one of the partners - and I would not distinguish physical health from emotional health - or in one of the children. Those are the three symptom locations of all families. Society is focused on the symptom locations instead of the emotional processes of the family. So the average is clear: if you got a problem in two you go to the third floor and if you have a problem in three you go to the fourth floor where they send you out if you have number one.

It is not that easy, it really is not.

The following is true. If you can promote in the family the differentiating factors that I mentioned before in the prophets you get to the symptom no matter where it is located. You don't have to be an expert on all the symptoms or any one symptom. If you can promote what I mentioned earlier out of four aspects of prophetic thinking you can get to the symptom wherever it is. The promoting of the prophetic elements as I just described, the promoting of differentiation as Mary Bowen has stated, has a broad spectrum. It will get you to the problem. But to do that the pastoral counsellor must work on that in his or her own life.

Those of us who have been teaching this way and training this way have now realized that the best form of supervision for any pastoral counsellor is getting them to go back and work on unresolved issues in their own family of origin. But that is far more significant than how they deal with any case. And that to the extent they can succeed at working with the anxious forces in their own family of origin, they do well with the families they are working with.

I'm running out of time, so there were certain other parts of this that I wanted to say. Instead what I want to end with is two stories to bring it all together and then I'm counting on the question period afterwards to develop some more of these ideas.

I'm going to tell you two stories. One involves a father, one involves a mother and it involves my effort to promote the prophetic element in each family.

The first family involves a father, a mother and three sons. The identified problem in the family has always been the oldest son, who is twenty years old. The parents' marriage has been incredibly successful, they don't fight, they love one another, they have good sex, they do things together and it is terrific. It is an interracial family. He is white and Jewish, she is black. They are both attorneys. The oldest son has constantly had problems with his life and the father has always worked hard to try to help this child. The son has blamed a lot of his problems on the fact that he is the son of an interracial marriage. He has never taken hold of his own destiny. He went off to college and in the second year dropped out under very mysterious circumstances. It is not clear which. He then started going to different institutions around the country, first to one for alcoholism. He claimed he was an alcoholic. Then he went to one for sexual dysfunction, claimed that that was his problem. Then he went to one for drug abuse.

The father who had the money would support the son. Nothing worked and the mother was unable to take stands at all and often would sabotage the father when he tried to take a stand. Father said that when he grew up he called his father every single day when he was in college, so that his relationship with his father was a very intense one. There it was positive intensity, here it is negative intensity. When the father married, his family almost cut him off because he married a black woman. But after the birth of this child everything got very good. So somehow or other this child's existence and life was part of the working out of everything within the family.

The father always tried to deal with the child reasonably. He always tried to deal with the child in his honest and upright way and what happened was, every time he did this the child took it, that is: the child took advantage of him. Finally one day I said to him: Would you be willing to write what I call a "straightening up letter" to your son? A straightening up letter is something I learned years ago. It is one in which the parent profiles himself to the child.

Well, he waited a bit and then the child called again and asked him to come out to help again, and he did not want to come out and see him a thousand miles away. The son did the usual thing of threatening to commit suicide. The father sat down and wrote the son the following letter. It was something like this.

Dear son,
I have spent a lot of time trying to help you out of all your problems. Nothing that I have ever done seems to have worked.
I am dead-up. If you wish to commit suicide, that is your choice. I just want you to know that if you do it, it certainly has not been in the tradition of our family issues. But the major thing I want you to understand is I will no longer be pulled down to your level of immaturity.

Within a week the son was home, still playing games, but father is now completely on a different side with this child and after years and years of all kinds of psychotherapy the son is beginning to show responsibility that he has never shown until the father made the change. Not because some therapist came up with the right idea, but because the father introduced what I call "the prophetic element" in here.

Those of us who worked this way have stopped seeing children. We will coach the parents instead. But now, let me tell you a completely other saga, still with the prophetic elements.

This involves a woman who is divorced from her husband and has four children. A son again, about twenty, who is just not doing anything with his life. A daughter, seventeen, who every time mother tries to straighten her out, simply gives her the finger. Twinboys, sixteen, on drugs and failing in highschool. There is a big cut off here. The father has almost nothing to do with the children.

I saw the mother, who is about fifty years old, for close to six months and nothing I said to her helped. No advice, no suggestions for strategy worked. Let me explain about this woman. She is fifty years old, Jewish, he is not. She works hard, she is kind of sexy but she has dish-pan hands. And there is something else about her. She rides a motorcycle. You will not find too many fifty-year old Jewish mothers who ride motorcycle. But she just loves it.

So one day I decided to work on the outrageous side of her. One day when she was complaining about things as usual, I said to her: Why don't you resign from motherhood, putting that in the paper and offer to trade your children in for a new Honda. She loved it. She went to her children and said: I quit. She called the father, who was eleven million dollars behind in child payments, and said: I'm giving you the children, I don't want to have anything to do with them.

A policewoman had to be called over to get the kids out of the house, after she signed a certain document. The oldest boy went to live with his father, the daughter went to live with some friends and the boys went into two different families. Her former husband called her and said: How could you do this to your own flesh and blood?

Her mother, seventy five years old and living in Florida, called her and said: isn't this being too hasty? Her older brother and a younger brother, in other words everybody in the family, tried to sabotage her, but she did it and she stayed with it. This occurred last December. She was dating a man much younger than she, who really was not good for her.

It is now eight months later and she has maintained this position all the way through. The son has, for the first time in his life, gone to work for his father. The daughter is about to enter college and keeps calling mother to find out if they can do things together. The sons are making a true school and the one who was pushing drugs has stopped. And mother has broken up with that man and is about to face life with a new sense of intension.

I just wanted to show you that it is possible to go in two entirely different directions in counselling, with that man taking a serious strong stay and this woman acting paradoxically and mischievously, and they are both manifestations of what I call the prophetic elements in pastoral counselling.

To repeat as a conclusion of what I stated:

One is the capacity to separate yourself out, but remain connected.
Two: be absolutely clear about where you stand.
Three: stay on course when others try to sabotage you and
Four: be outrageous when it is necessary in the name of God.

'Subham', The Concept of Wholeness in Pastoral Counselling in The Hindu Cultural Context

Padmasani J. Gallup

Confronted culture

Contemporary Indian culture reflects its millenia-old Hindu religious history. It continues to be characterised by caste hierarchy, subservience to authority, insularity and resistance to change, and ritualism, among other factors. Indian society has been challenged to change, confronted by a system of public education brought by Western trading powers and offered to all, by the process of modernization consequent to rapid adaptation of Western science and technology, and by the awakening of hitherto oppressed and suppressed members within that society. Western formal education intruded into the Hindu socio-religious context with explosive ideas and ideology. Based on Christian conceptions of person-hood and on convictions about the equality and preciousness of each individual, it faced a belief-system in which persons were ordered in a vertical, high-low, hierarchy in which all human effort was to be expended in the pursuit of *moksa* for the male members - the union of the human soul (*atman*) with the all-pervading *Brahman*. Straight-away this education was a challenge to traditional acceptance of inequality and called persons to corporate responsibility.

One of the outcomes of this confrontation can be perceived in the psychosocial problems of everyday living faced by a number of persons. In order to identify issues for contextual counselling, we may begin with a brief outline of the Hindu view of the person, proceed to look at three recent incidents and their possible resolution, and examine the Hindu

understanding of the goals of human endeavour for some clues to the
search for wholeness.

Hindu view of the person

Hinduism, the religion of eightyfive percent of India's people, is non-
credal: anyone can be a Hindu. As a religion, it is a way of life following
certain laws, practices and rituals based on a hierarchical social structure.
Purpose and meaning in life is to be found in the journey toward *moksa*
of the *atman* of every male Hindu. This journey may take a number of
rebirths. Souls of women may attain *moksa* as they are reborn as males.
The laws governing individual and social life are set out in the *dharma* for
each; dharma is variously interpreted as 'moral duty', 'law', or 'right
action'.

Over the centuries these laws have taken on a conserving rigidity which
is almost impossible to change. Each person's *dharma* is proscribed within
in limits of *desa* (country: cultural setting), *kala* (past and present history
of cultural setting), *shrama* (the particular stage of life within the cycle of
births) and *guna* (genetic, psycho-biological make-up).

The individual male is expected to develop along certain set ideals toward
the ultimate goal. These ideals are articulated as psychosocial *ashramadharma* stages of life. Childhood is not recognized as a formal stage.
Specific attitudes and behaviour are prescribed for each stage with
personal and social implications. The *Brahmacharya* - student, 'adolescent', prepares himself to become a *grahastha* - married head of a house,
caring for the poor and the weak. After fulfilling his *dharma* in this stage,
he moves on to become a *vanaprastha* (literally, 'forest-dweller') to begin
the process of withdrawal from worldly care and attachments - finally
realizing in the last, *sanyasa* stage, total withdrawal and concentration on
devotional and other exercises toward the attainment of *moksa*. All other
creatures and persons subserve this psychosocial development of the
Hindu male.

The *dharma* of each person is prescribed according to his place in the caste hierarchy. Women's *dharma* is mainly to serve the men and other family members in order to earn merit to be born as a male.

A not untypical modern, adult, Indian male

Kumar, a forty-plus government employee has a wife, Kala, a daughter, Jaya aged seven, and a three year old son, Vimal - apparently an ideal, attractive Christian family. But, Kala, a competent college lecturer, poured out a narrative of acts of mental and physical violence perpetrated on her and the children by Kumar over a span of years. Typically, Kumar would return home very late at night, having enjoyed an evening with friends or at a movie. He would wake the sleeping children because he "wanted to enjoy talking with them". Kala would have to prepare a fresh, hot dinner and wait on him while he ate. He never told her where he had been or what he had done. When he was full and sleepy, he would retire to bed regardless of the wakefulness of the others. He did not comprehend that there was anything amiss in his pattern of behaviour. These were the least offensive of his actions. He had no hesitation about beating and abusing his wife and children. Kala had had enough, and wondered what her options were for a safe and quiet life.

The problem of Kumar may be identified as that of one who had not resolved the unconscious feelings of anger toward his mother. The mother happens to be another 'typical case'. She exerted such a pathological control over Kumar, her first-born, that she used to brush his teeth for him even up to age eleven! The issue seems to be the complex one of the so-called "passive" Indian woman safeguarding her own fragile ego by manipulating the male under her control. Her husband, inordinately proud of his son, indulged him to the extent that he never had a want, nor, one would suspect, any freedom to grow to be himself. Without freedom, he had not learned any responsibility, either. He took what he wanted, expected those around him to serve him, was filled with unrecognized rage against his mother, and took it out on his wife.

Search for wholeness in the mutuality of partnership - woman's status in Hindu culture

Hindu culture has allowed only a dependent identity for women. Some women live in relative peace and contentment, accepting and adjusting to this role. Those who have been absorbed in finding and providing the basic necessities for bringing up a family have developed the ego-strength of the survivor. Middle-class, educated and economically independent women have faced the need for a consciously independent identity for themselves and have often developed into stable adult personalities. Those who have not managed to appropriate independent identities adopt pathological strategies of control, especially of their sons. It is painfully true to those wives whose husbands act out their unacknowledged rage against their mothers by abusing their wives. A vicious spiral results, of seeking identity through overt or covert control over those seen as weak or lesser beings, (e.g., servants). However, Kala is attempting to break this spiral and is anxious to relate 'normally' to her husband and children. The origin of the pathological relationship may be traced to some extent to the Hindu world-view which presumes the supremacy of the adult male. The expectation that all others are to serve the ultimate goal of the Hindu male legitimizes his use of others for the fulfilment of his wishes and desires. This can reach pathological dimensions of self-centredness and cause severe problems in relationships within a family. In joint family situations, the status of the grandfather is that of either a benevolent or tyrannical patriarch. Grown sons have to take on sub-servient attitudes. The evolution of a pecking order in order to assume an identity is inevitable, with the attendant risk of hidden resentments.

Reinterpretation of Hindu mythology

What is the task of pastoral counselling in the case of Kala? She could be encouraged to look at mythological heroines who undertake the task of bringing about change in situations of conflict. Indian mythology narrates stories about women who emerge with strong identities in spite of all manner of vicissitudes; Sita, Savitri and Kannagi are such heroines.

Damayanthi is one such. Her husband, Nalan, whom she herself chose among all the princes who had attended her *swayamvaram*,[1] turns out to be a gambler with wanderlust. After losing even the clothes off his back, he leaves Damayanthi, taking half of her sari to cover his nakedness. She returns to her father's house, but cannot rest. She organizes a second *swayamvaram* and chooses the same Nalan, because, without a husband she cannot have sons to earn moksa for her, which is her only salvation. Her *dharma* dictates this. But she, being stronger and the more mature, becomes the rescuer, saving Nalan from his own folly so that he, too, can fulfil his *dharma*. Likewise, Kala must work out her own salvation by not only serving Kumar, but also by helping him to change his unacceptable behaviour. Hindu culture, while giving a low status to woman, elevates her to the status of a goddess (a giver) in the family as wife and mother.

A wife is half the man transcends
In value for all other friends.
She every earthly blessing brings,
And even redemption from her springs.
In lovely homes, companions bright,
These charming women give delight;
Like fathers wise, in duty tried,
To virtuous acts they prompt and guide.
Whenever we suffer pain and grief
Like mothers kind they bring relief.

Mahabharata[2]

A father excels ten upadhyayas (teachers)
in glory,
But a mother excels a thousand fathers.

Manu[3]

---

1   The ancient practice of allowing the daughter of a wealthy citizen to choose her
     husband through publicly garlanding him in the company of a number of suitors.
2   Hindu epic poem of 1000 B.D. (A.C.E.)
3   Codifier of Hindu law of 2 Century A.D.

This status-augmentation can be utilized to strengthen Kala in counselling. Counselling may encourage Kala to try to win Kumar over through patience and thoughtful care to evoke a sense of responsibility and a desire to be a partner in life. She must be cautioned against perpetuating the vicious spiral, and helped to deal constructively with her frustrations. Pastoral counselling would stress the equality of men and women in creation, the mutuality of giving and receiving of care and love; it would recall the need to be a 'house-holder' loving and caring for the young and weak. Kumar cannot be left in lonely splendour, but through a saving partnership of respect, through verbal and non-verbal communication husband and wife have to seek their good through responsible parenthood, released from unrealistic expectations of themselves and of each other. Kala does not wish to leave her husband. A separated or divorced woman is as full of bitterness as a widow. She is blamed, ostracised and cursed. Counselling is directed toward achieving the ideal wholeness of male-female partnership as visioned in the Arthanareesvara union of Siva and Parvathi, gods of Hindu Saivaism. It is sometimes referred to as the union of Sivam and Sakti = goodness and power. In this search for wholeness the whole family, aunts, uncles, cousins etc. could be involved.

A college student: youth or adult

A young college junior was elected to the office of Secretary of the students' union. Straightaway he went to the women's hostel and announced that he would lead a strike as soon as the new academic year commenced. He saw no need to identify an issue for such 'direct action'.

Such a bid for revolt can be recognised as a pathetic cry for recognition or notice. It can be seen as part of the ultimate search for identity, and an acceptable world-view.

For a number of college students the transition from a rural, simple, basic style of life to urban sophistication is discomfiting if not shattering. From identity as a youngster dependent on parents and other elders in the village family, he is thrust willy-nilly into the role of budding expert or authority on world affairs, politics, economics, the sciences and tech-nology. He is often forced into a position of responsibility and decision-making for which his psychological development has not prepared him. Even if he hails from an urban, middle-class family, sometimes this same situation obtains, especially if he is the first to attain university education. Relating to women becomes a behavioural issue in a co-educational institution for those brought up on strict taboos. Some rural and urban families do not allow brothers and sisters to have any normal sibling relationship after puberty. Some cannot even converse. The adolescent's awakening sexuality is rudely and pathologically suppressed and seeks outlets in unacceptable ways. The cultural ideal being abstinence or sex controlled toward procreation, (Ramanujam, p.52), there is much guilt. "Masturbation and seminal emission are still believed to cause psychia-tric disorders." (Venkoba Rao, p.301). This causes a split in value-orien-tation; the ideal being so far removed from experience.

Education in today's India becomes a factor in the confusion of youth. While rural or urban middle-class ethos and social norms are founded on the stringent hierarchy of caste division, a student in the university is challenged to adopt consciously a life-style and attitude of equality. While his family assures him a status and position due to birth alone, away from his family he is told that he has to earn his status through hard work. In the dormitory a brahmin may well share sleeping quarters, dining and toilet facilities with an 'untouchable'. This may give rise to identity and role confusion. Role refusal results when freedom is pursued without its concomitant of responsibility in a situation where the youngster cannot identify 'responsible living'. He is also bombarded by differing and seduc-tive ideologies. He may give in to fatalism.

Hindu cultural ethos, however, engenders a mind set which manages to assume normal functioning in spite of contradictions. Compartmentaliza-tion is a coping mechanism adopted by the Indian psyche. Moreover, as Sudhir Kakar has identified, primary process thinking prevails among the young as well as adults, allowing the mind to hold contradictions together without causing psychic disorientation. (Kakar, 1978).

Search for holistic world-view and viable identity

It is fairly well recognized that the Indian bio-social structure has not recognized adolescence as a developmental stage. Rites of passage observed formally, and sometimes with pomp and ceremony, at puberty for both boys and girls, mark the end of childhood and entrance into the adult world of work and responsibility. Both boys and girls had been indulged and surrounded with warmth and affection as children. Now the young boy is required to take his place with the men, in the fields and elsewhere and be gainfully employed. The young girl leaves innocent playfulness, joins the women in their subservient functions, is constrained to guard her chastity most vigilantly, and becomes a care-giver. There is neither the leisure nor the stimulus to begin to reflect about 'Who am I' or 'What am I'. Most youngsters accept an imposed identity. Perhaps this is why the Hindu adult male seems constrained to devote energy and time in an attempt at self-realization in late adulthood and old age.

In psychosocial development in Western cultures, adolescence is a distinct stage during which the search for an identity predominates. The crisis of this stage, according to Erikson, is 'identity' versus 'identity confusion' and the virtue is 'fidelity'. (Childhood and Society).

Sudhir Kakar relates this stage and the preceding one of school age to the two parts of the first *ashramadharma*, that of brahmacharya:

> ... *in which the school child, growing into youth, learned the basic skills relevant to his future adult working role, while he lived together with other students and the guru... The task... I would say, lies in the knowing of one's dharma, which could consist of acquiring the skills in one's caste and in winning identity based on a caste identity and the identification with and emulation of the guru.*
>
> (Identity and Adulthood, 'Setting the Stage', p.7)

This is the ancient ideal. In today's world it is not possible. While a young student may manage to hold together the contradictions of a casteless campus life-style and Hindu family ethos of strict caste observance, he/she still has to know who she/he is.

An equally serious issue is a viable world-view to which the youngster can be committed. The Hindu world-view is necessarily crumbling as India gets catapulted into a world capitalist economy from a rural-based barter system, and into a technology-dominated world. India is rapidly being sucked into the global village. Its youth is challenged to make meaningful life in this global village where nuclear warheads have been stockpiled with the potential of blowing up the whole planet earth; where neutron bombs will spare the Taj Mahal but will not leave any living being to enjoy it; where bomb-making has been made as simple, and maybe as satisfying, as assembling a tinker-toy structure for an elementary school child. Modernization and dependence on technology has given rise to a sense of helplessness or powerlessness and man becomes less important than machine. There is no place for God among the technocrats. Rapid nuclearization of the tried and true joint family structure and the breaking apart of rural culture based on Hindu religion marks the erosion of traditional institutions and indicates a shaking of the foundations.

Consequently, young persons in college are confused and cynical. There is no 'identification with and emulation of the guru'. Their professors do not practice what they profess. Yet, the youngsters do hunger for a *guru-sishya* (master-disciple) relationship; they want ideals and seek for leaders with power and charisma. The only power they encounter may be that of violence and terror; there is no grace. Or they get sucked into fatalism.

Counselling in this context for confused, leaderless young persons may have to adopt the directive approach of the rational-emotive type. Leading the youngsters to search in their superego, they may find a residue of the moral and ethical teachings of the ancients. They can be encouraged to examine their own literature to recapture the idealism and ethical norms of a viable world view. (E.g. the couplets of the *Tirukkural*, on right daily living based on charity, love and peace.)

Venkoba Rao suggests the use of the *Bhagavadgita*, which offers "the concept of total surrender, eagerness of the pupil to enlighten himself,

liberty to interrogate intelligently, desire for knowledge to dispel igno-
rance, and absence of coercion on the part of [the counsellor]." (Rao, in
Transcultural Psychiatry, John J. Cox, Ed, p.302). The disciplines of yoga
may be introduced at this age so that students may freely choose the path
most suited to them. While encouraging the young persons to pursue
freedom at this stage, they should be helped to accept responsibility as
the other side of the coin. They soon shall acquire the *ashrama* of
householder and care-giver, and must be prepared.

There can be a viable identity as a human, an Indian, without the
constrictions of casteism and communalism. The human is to be understood in the wholeness of body, mind and spirit without the guilt associated with sexuality. The Christian acceptance of human beings as created
in God's image includes physiological, psychological and spiritual enti-
ties. To assist the youngsters to accept this and work toward such an
identity is the task of pastoral counselling. Search for wholeness will be
integrating self-identity with a viable world view. At this age young
women and men are keen on ecological concerns. The Indian view of the
spark of the divine in each created being could help in articulating
environmental concerns, and corporate responsibility.

Self immolation and the quest for identity

Consequent to the recent shatteringly tragic death of former Indian
Prime Minister Rajiv Gandhi, seventeen deaths by suicide were reported,
and it is recognized that several more went unreported. When the late
Chief Minister of Tamil Nadu, M.G. Ramachandran fell seriously ill, no
less than thirty-five persons took their own lives, and when he died,
several more souls joined his departed one. A number of these suicides
were young adults, but nearly a third were between thirty-five and fifty
years of age, both men and women.

The universal human need for recognition is exaggerated in these persons. Their identity is cathected to the charismatic leader and the ego is
not individuated in a 'normal' psychosocial development.

Ramanujam, observing that adolescence is an urban phenomenon brought on partly by West-aping advertising media, suggests that in the Indian psycho-cultural context one could posit the concept of extended adolescence into adult years.

> *If we accept the thesis that conflicts appropriate to a particular phase of development should be resolved, at least to some extent, before moving on to the next stage, it is understandable that since a culture does not recognize adolescence as a distinct phase, no provision is made to facilitate the resolution of such conflicts. It is only natural that these conflicts should be seen in adulthood.*
>
> (Kakar, 79, p. 49).

Again, when a person is at the bottom of the hierarchical social pyramid of caste, the message received is: "you are nothing, unclean, unworthy, unwanted."

Women and outcastes often internalize this message, accepting this non-identity. The only way to acquire the ego-strength necessary for normal human interaction is to be attached to some other strong ego in utter dependency. A psychological need to be noticed may drive such persons to self-immolation - it is always undertaken in public. Not only is there recognition: but since the act is connected to the death of a charismatic leader, his glory may spill over onto these persons. Young adults may resort to this 'last act' in a frenzy of grief, as the frustration of unemployment, confusion as to who they are and what their place is in the world around them reaches a peak and throws them over. Such persons have no learned means to work through their anguish of separation or frustration.

Search for an adult maturity

Counselling for persons unable to deal with the great loss of identity suffered at the death of the charismatic figure may use Hindu ideas of union and separation. While the pantheistic belief of the Hindu encourages a feeling of oneness with all matter, animate and inanimate, it also recognizes the independent and individual entity of *atman* in each living being. The *dharma* of each *atman* is to seek its liberation through the fulfilment of set duties toward one's self and others. The sense of duty is strongly imprinted in the Hindu psyche. Counselling may attempt to turn the dependency identified from the human figures toward God and self. Using the concept of 'separate yet fused' that is part of the marriage rite, could begin the process. Techniques of meditation and self-hypnosis could be taught in order to internalize the affirmation 'I am a child of God; I am worthy'. The path of *Bakhti yoga* could be utilized to explore dependence and independence. The sense of duty may be utilized to help lead useful and independent lives.

India's contribution to the search for wholeness

Perhaps a significant contribution of Indian culture is that it takes religion seriously. Every aspect of life, every prescribed duty, is learned within the framework of Hindu religion. The most greedy entrepreneur, the most corrupt politician, will begin his day with *puja* (worship) at the household shrine, (or his wife does it on his behalf). Being in touch, however remotely, with the source of Being keeps the heart and mind on an even keel. Guilt is not a burden as heavy as experienced in Christendom, because the Hindu system acknowledges repeated chances through the cycle of births for working out one's *dharma*, for making amends and for atonement.

The negative aspect of this religious foundation for all of life's rituals is that it becomes forced and unnatural, even inhuman. This is why Mahatma Gandhi, a staunch Hindu, accepted the teachings of Jesus as possessing universal applicability, and the stalwarts who hammered out the constitution for the socialist republic of India insisted that it be strictly secular while adopting a number of principles from the Biblically-influenced constitution of the United States of America.

Exercises such as meditation and the different systems of yoga are meant to enable the individual to attain adult maturity. Concepts of adulthood are integral to the Hindu world view, which seeks to give meaning to life.

Since the world image focuses on liberation of the atman, two stages of adulthood are posited: one to fulfil all the dharma of living in the world with others in a variety of relationships; the next, a conscious withdrawal from all worldly attachments and preparation for ultimate union with Brahman in death. As Kakan observes, the healthy adult of western understanding, (derived from psychoanalysis of pathological persons), is "only a prelude to the liberated adult. Ideally adulthood does not stop at prudence, but must lead towards liberation." ('Relative Realities' in Identity and Adulthood, p.123).

Hindu culture and philosophy has assumed that there is a higher order of knowledge (*vidhya*) available to humans which will lead them to liberation beyond nature and radically different from physical, sensory knowledge (*avidhya*). It has evolved four systems of *yoga* as disciplines which will lead to this *vidhya* and consequent liberation.

1. *Karma yoga* does not require physical withdrawal, but enjoins activity which is disinterested and detached; activity according to the *ashrama* of the householder for the care of others.
2. *Bakhti yoga* is the path of pure devotion leading to the spirituality of total dependence on the godhead and forgetfulness of the physical self.
3. *Gnana yoga* furnishes knowledge through intellectual exercise of meditation and mental practices.
4. *Raja yoga* utilizes psycho-physiological techniques to transform the habitual modes of experiencing. Through intense concentration a feeling of oneness with the objects of creation is achieved as well as a heretofore unknown intensity of awareness.

All of these paths lead to the detachment necessary for leaving this earthly life gracefully, in a realistic and natural acceptance of the inevitable. They may also take the individual beyond this initial purpose to an 'exaltation' beyond all human imaginings, to the *samadhi* and *santhi* of total union in *moksa*. *Santhi* is a concept of wholeness, of full integration of mind, body and spirit offered through the yogic systems of hard discipline that Hindu culture can offer for all persons. The whole yogic journey can be interpreted as the way that the self escapes isolation and the finality of death through identification on a grand, universal scale, with the universe of matter and spirit.

Contextual counselling in India aims toward adult maturity and takes seriously the Hindu world view, expectations, goals and liberative principals, adapting, countering, and working through them in response to individual needs.

Pastoral counselling brings in the Christian concern for the wholeness, the blessed well-being of all persons. It would seek to counteract the fatalism and indifference, which arises out of the Hindu world view, toward human suffering and the powers of evil. At the same time it would search for aspects that would help to bring wholeness in the Hindu culture.

Much of this paper is conceptual. The case of Kala is the one in process now. It is hoped that counsellors in India could try these concepts and evolve others to bring wholeness to suffering and hurting persons. It is also hoped that the place of the faith community in this endeavour and search for wholeness in pastoral counselling would be explored by others. We Indians are community oriented, not individualistic as Western people tend to be. Cross-cultural counselling could use community as an agent for bringing wholeness, the *subham* of blessedness.

Bibliography

1. Kakar, Sudhir, Ed., *Identity and Adulthood,* Oxford University Press, Delhi, 1979.
   Kakar, Sudhir, Ed., *The inner World*, A Psychoanalytic Study of Childhood and Society in India, O.U.P., Delhi, 1978.

2. Erikson, Eric, *Childhood and Society,* Faber and Faber, London, 1961.
   Erickson, Eric, *Identity: Youth and Crisis*, W.W. Norton, New York, 1968.

3. Cox, John, Ed., *Transcultural Psychiatry*, Croom Helm, London, 1986.

4. Belkin, Gary S., *Introduction to Counselling*, Wm. C. Brown, Publishers, Dubuque, 1988.

5. Pedersen, Paul B.; Draguns, Juris G.; Lonner, Walter J.; Trimble, Joseph E., *Counselling Across Cultures*, University of Hawaii press, Honolulu, 1989.

6. Srinivas, M.N., *The Changing Position of Indian Women*, O.U.P., New Delhi, 1978.

7. Spratt, Philip, *Hindu Culture and Personality*, Manaktalas, Bombay, 1966.

8. Sue, Deral W., *Counselling the Culturally Different*, John Wiley & Sons, New York, 1981.

9. Sen Gupta, S, *Women in Indian Folklore: A Survey of Social Status and Position*, Indian Publications, Calcutta, 1969.

10. Ross, Aileen D., *The Hindu Family in its Urban Setting*. Univ. of Toronto Press, Toronto, 1961.

11. Radhakrishnan, Sarvapalli, *The Hindu View of Life*, Macmillan, New York, 1929.

12. Munroe, Ruth, *Cross-Cultural Human Development*, J. Aronson, New York, 1975.

13. Kapur, Promilla, *The Changing Status of the Working Woman in India*. Vikas Publications. Delhi, 1974.

14. Dimmitt, Cornelia; van Buitenen, J.A.B., *Classical Hindu Mythology*, Temple Univ. Press, Philadelphia, 1979.

Devouring Mother or Wounded Healer?
Liberating New Models of Caring in Feminist Theology

Mary Grey

Introduction

There is an ancient Greek fable, retold by the German philosopher, Heidegger: *'The Myth of Care'*

> *"Once when 'Care' was crossing a river, she saw some clay; she thought-fully took up a piece and began to shape it. While she was meditating on what she had made, Jupiter came by. 'Care' asked Him to give it spirit, and this he gladly granted. But when she wanted her name to be bestowed upon it, he forbade this, and demanded that it be given his name instead. While 'Care' and Jupiter were disputing, Earth rose and desired that her own name be bestowed upon the creature, since she had furnished it with part of her body. They asked Saturn to be their arbiter, and he made the following decision, which seemed a just one: "Since you, Jupiter, have given it spirit, you shall receive that spirit at its death; and since you, Earth, have given its body, you shall receive that body. But since 'Care' first shaped this creature, she shall possess it as long as she lives. And because there is now a dispute among you as to its name, let it be called 'homo', for it is made out of 'humus' (earth).'"*[1]

Heidegger told this story to highlight the primordial, ontological significance of 'Care' for human existence. In this primal sense 'Care' is not a virtue, to be arbitrarily exercised by benevolent individuals, or because one feels sorry for the old or less fortunate: care is the very pre-condition for human existence, growth, and meaningful relating. So being 'care-ful' is not simply how we look after money and possessions, but the quality of commitment to ongoing forms of life on our planet. To be 'care-less', 'care-free', is to separate and isolate oneself from this pulsating heart of meaning. 'Care' is not a free-floating emotion or ethical charge: it must be interpreted and structured again and again according to the historical, political and social context. What follows is an attempt to contextualise 'Care' from a feminist theological perspective.

I will begin with the theological context of *'Women-Church'*: what does 'care' mean within this context? Secondly, I will bring a gender analysis to bear on the way care has been interpreted within the Christian tradition, summed up, above all, by the spirituality of motherhood. Thirdly, within a feminist ethics of care and responsibility I will develop new models of caring which enable 'Care' to once again be the creative energy which stimulates growth - both spiritual and physical - and healing, in a broken world.

1. What is our context?

Feminist theology has arisen in response to the discrimination and oppression of women in society and Church. In many cases this is a triple, interlocking, discrimination - of race, sex and class, requiring specific analysis and agenda according to the cultural situation. The discrimination against most white women in N. Europe is on a different scale from that of Asian and African women in many parts of the world - and in Europe itself. Yet Feminist theology is a theology of liberation, committed to the liberation of all women: "Till all women are free, no woman is free!" is an oft-repeated slogan.

Secondly, the focus here is on the consequences of the structures of caring for which *Christian Theology itself* is responsible: so the fact that women are absent from these founding structures is the first problem. (By 'founding structures' I mean the dominant theological interpretations of Scripture, doctrine and ethics as well as the absence of women - until comparatively recently - from official ordained ministry and decision-making bodies. Clearly this has certain ecumenical variations across the denominations). If we wanted a scriptural image to encapsulate this, we can focus on Hagar, the concubine of Abraham (Genesis 16 and 21). She is eclipsed by the dominant structures in terms of 'inferior' race - she was Egyptian not Jewish, oppressed in terms of class - she was a slave, and inferior in terms of gender - she was female and sexually an object to be used by Abraham. And yet she was one of the first mothers of a promised child, who received a revelation from God:

"You are with child and shall bear a son.
You shall name him Ishmael." (Gen. 16.12)

What is more, Hagar - in contrast with others in the Bible - lived on to tell others about her Divine vision:

"Have I indeed seen God and lived after the vision?" (Gen. 16.14)

And yet, it is Sarah, wife of the patriarch, whom we remember as central to our tradition. Hagar remains on the margins.

The point to stress is that even though women are present to the tradition, it is either as outsider in terms of exclusion from positions of authority, or as included in terms of usefulness, and as needing to be defined and controlled by men; but never as equal partners, capable of self-definition. Here theology has rested on analyses of human subjectivity of philosophy and psychology which define the human being in male terms, and strayed far from the original insight that both man and woman are created in the image of God (Genesis 1.17).

Thirdly, moving to the contemporary context: we live in a culture of violence, a culture which is in love with violence, which even eroticises violence and systematizes crucifixions. How often do you hear, whenever altruism or idealism vanishes, the cry "we need a good war, to bring out the best in people(!)?" This culture of violence covers both public expressions like war, and now football vandalism, as well as sexual attacks on women and children both publicly and domestically. We live at a time, when it is now possible to speak openly about the level of domestic sexual abuse - both battering and incest - and to make the links between this and the structures of religion.[2] (Later I will link this with structures of caring).

For all these reasons it is essential to affirm that *'Women are Church'*, the People of God - even if invisible in the founding contract, and that the context of being woman, outsider, defined and controlled by others, our experience alien to the dominant one, demands its own pastoral care and ministry. This is why 'Woman-Church' has come into being. Far from seeking to be 'a Church' as an institution, an organization, in the accepted sense of the words, 'Woman-Church' seeks to be Church liberated from patriarchy. It seeks the dismantling of clericalism and the distorted power structures of patriarchy which keep women forever outsiders. Yet it is no breakaway movement - most women who are involved and inspired by its aims attempt to transform structures of traditional Church, from their marginal position, on the strength of their conviction that 'Women are Church'. I will now explore the meaning of Woman-Church in 3 ways, before asking what are the ethics and structures of care which this new ecclesiology inspires.

First, Woman-Church is, as Rosemary Ruether has said, an Exodus community, that is, a community in Exodus from patriarchal oppression of society and Church:

> *"We are not in exile, but the Church is in exile with us. Holy Wisdom, the Mother-face of God has fled with us from the high thrones of patriarchy and has gone into Exodus with us."*[3]

This image of being in the Wilderness, nourished by milk and honey, but still dispossessed from the Promised Land, is complemented by Elizabeth Schüssler-Fiorenza's definition of Woman-church as a community of equals. Woman-Church, she wrote, "seeks to name theologically the alienation, anger, pain, dehumanization engendered by sexism and racism in society and Church."[4] It seeks to call the entire Church to conversion and repentance. For this task the Bible is indeed the book of Woman-Church: but instead of allowing this to be used against women, we now read it with a four-fold feminist hermeneutical interpretation.

First, with a *hermeneutic of suspicion* which assumes that the Biblical texts are androcentric and serve patriarchal functions. Secondly, a *hermeneutics of proclamation* will elucidate the texts which actually serve to chain women in oppression - like saying to a battered woman that she must take up her Cross daily just as Jesus did; at the same time it will highlight for proclaiming in Church and liturgy the texts which transcend their androcentric background and announce a liberating vision. Thirdly, a *hermeneutic of remembrance* proposes new models of interpretation which bring women from the background to the centre of the biblical community. Thus we are allowed a glimpse of womens' leadership in early Christianity and theology. But we will also keep alive the 'memoria passionis' - the memory of suffering and struggles of women. Finally, a *hermeneutic of creative actualization* seeks to re-tell the stories from a feminist perspective of liberation, (rather as I tried to re-claim the story of Hagar for Woman-Church).

More recently, Elizabeth Schüssler Fiorenza has developed these ideas in recognition of the different cultures and contexts of women. She calls Woman-Church "a bounded open space", where there are overlapping communities and discourses. The openness means our openness to listening, understanding and ministering to each other. The *boundedness* consists both in recognising the 'otherness' and differences of language, culture, race and class. 'Boundedness' too means a distancing from all that oppresses and does not liberate. And this brings me to the *ethical* dimension of Woman-Church. This is given prominence by Mary Hunt, (another American feminist theologian, who founded WATER, Womens' Alliance for Theology, Ethics and Ritual). She sees Woman-Church in a loosely-defined way as groups of women and men, who, as justice-seeking friends, break together word and sacrament. Thus all definitions ground themselves in the struggle against oppression as basis for the ecclesia of women. But struggle in itself has never been a sufficient definition of Church. The root meaning of 'ecclesia' is a 'Gathering-together': in the Christian sense this is realised in celebration of God's saving actings in Christ. Woman-Church *can* celebrate - despite the continuing pain and suffering of women - because it is incarnating a Christian vision of love and freedom for our times, and for our people, and because it believes that God's healing and redeeming actions are revealing themselves in the poorest of the poor. Thus the structures of caring of 'Woman-Church' are the context for what I develop here. This I would like to call the basis for an ethics of Woman-Church.

The problem I discuss can be put in a nutshell: 'Care' and 'caring' - expressed above all in 'Love for neighbour' - are the very keynote of the Christian ethics and the ethics of the Kingdom of God. Self-denial, 'losing self only to find it' are frequently cited as accompanying exhortations. Yet - as I hinted above - this ethic has often trapped women in cycles of misery, in wretched marriages, domestic violence, in unequal work distribution, in acceptance of lower paid or despised kinds of work, in the loss of career through care for children and elderly relatives, in being idealised as tender nurturers, while at the same time dying from having too many children or working long hours in factories. In famine and disaster situations in Third world countries it is the women and children who die in greatest numbers, and with women one factor is that their energy and concern goes to feeding their families. They are themselves the last to eat.

My question is: in the context of Woman-Church which I have defined as 'women ministering in mutuality', how could we come to an ethic of care which was liberating for women - yet at the same time faithful to the Gospel message.

2. 'Devouring mother or wounded healer'?

The most approved-of way for women to enter the social contract - or be part of society - has traditionally by being mothers. 'Become anonymous to propagate the species!' has been the command given to women - and this command has crossed all cultures until, comparatively recently, family planning offered a degree of choice to women. (But this choice has scarcely ever been free, but was itself dependent on money, religion and the cooperation of husband or partner). Sociologically speaking, the father represents 'sign' and 'time': "in the name of the Father" literally sums up the way society organizes its institutions and inheritance.[5]

Transcendence is masculine, guaranteed by a God predominantly symbolised as male. Immanence is static and female. Spiritually speaking, motherhood has been encouraged ostensibly because it was supposed to sum up the 'quintessence of what it meant to be a woman', and secondly, because it was a living icon of the Gospel ideal of Christian self-giving love or 'agape'. That this is still so - in the Roman Catholic circles at least - can be shown by a quotation from the Apostolic Letter of Pope John Paul II, *Mulieris Dignitatem* (1984):

> *"Motherhood implies from the beginning a special openness to the new person: and this is precisely the woman's 'part': in this openness, in conceiving and giving birth to a child, the woman 'discovers herself through a sincere gift of self'... Scientific analysis confirms that the very physical constitution of women is naturally disposed to motherhood... At the same time this also corresponds to the psycho-physical structure of women... Motherhood is linked to the personal structure of the woman and to the personal dimension of the gift"*.[6](Underline in original)

Now it is far from the case that a feminist analysis wants in any way to undermine the importance of motherhood, especially here, when my hope is to uncover juster models of care. My concern is both that this definition is essentialist and confining for women - in restricting their 'true being' to motherhood, and, secondly, that it serves to gloss over the suffering of women as mothers.

Think of the 'Pietà' of Michelangelo - the icon of 'Mater Dolorosa', the 'Stabat Mater' of sacred song. How this has summed up the grief of countless mothers who - since Mary stood by the Cross - have mourned the sons destroyed by military conflict. The mother, reservoir of all pain. Maria Assumpta, the mother, promise of Resurrection - as consolation for the cutting-short of this life. The tears of the Virgin-Mother as giving the only permitted Christian expression to female exuberant sexuality, so channelled and controlled by patriarchy. The discourse of Mary represents the limits of societal expression for Christian womanhood. And sometimes I think nothing will ever change, haunted as we are today by pictures of skeletal mothers with dying babies - from Ethiopia, Iraq, Bangladesh, Kurdistan, and so on. So frequently do these pictures appear

on our television screens, that I despair now of their power to change us
at all.

But what has this to do with Christian theological categories? The danger
is, first, that in stressing the salvific value of suffering as the preferred
way of following Jesus, that we have encouraged a mystique of suffering
which has blinded us to injustice and oppression.[7] The core of the
Christian ethic is seen to be 'dying to self' in order to love others in a
selfless way. But women are socialised into caring for others from childhood: and this is a cross-cultural phenomenon. Recently in Amsterdam
Central Station I saw a 9 year-old girl cuddling a doll. Her mother was
annoyed because she lavished so much attention on this doll. My mind
flashed back to India, where I had been a few weeks earlier. Just such
attention by girls the same age had been lavished on real babies -
sometimes more than one at the same time. There the child takes over as
primary caretaker where the real mother is working on the fields. So
central is caring to the identity of women - a caring which can easily
replace child, for husband, for sick person, elderly relative and so on -
that there is a real danger that a strong sense of self is never developed.
Rather, a blurred, or mediated sense of self is more likely - which is not
quite sure where the boundaries of self are constituted.[8] Hence the loss
or breakdown of a relationship can mean a real loss of self. Even more
serious, where Christianity commands its followers to 'lose yourself in
order to find it', in many cases there is *no* self to be lost. A woman can
become a 'mediated self', defined in relation to child, husband, parent,
religious superior, and therefore almost destroyed by the death or departure of any of these.

The second reason for confronting the structures of theology is that its
understanding of sin and guilt have often held women responsible for
failures in caring. Because of the tradition of blaming women for the Fall,
(Genesis 3.16), a greater burden is placed on women for the moral fibre
of society. The stereotype of woman as temptress and witch has haunted
our tradition. Moreover women are held responsible for the welfare of
children - and husband - and themselves assume the guilt when things go
wrong.

And thirdly, there is a direct link between this responsibility for sin and motherhood which focusses on female sexuality. If we think of the teaching of the 1st Letter to Timothy,

> *"For Adam was created first, and Eve afterward; and it was not Adam who was deceived; it was the woman who, yielding to deception, fell into sin. Yet she will be saved through motherhood..."* (1 Tim 3.16),

we can see how strong the pressures on women have been to accept motherhood as God-given role which at the same time had an atoning significance. There is still at least an *implicit* belief in the expiatory quality of the pains of childbirth and sorrows of motherhood.[9]

But there is another factor at play. And I think this is the key to the problem. For the icon of the Christian Mother, Virginal Mother, Mater Dolorosa, hides the older archetype of mother, Magna Mater, Earth Mother, the Great Mother goddess figures of Egypt, Babylon, Greece, Rome, and within Canaan itself.[10] The discourse of Christian motherhood has needed to be severely controlled because the symbolism of the Great Mother seemed so terrifying. Now, (perhaps too late?) we realise what we have lost, what we have destroyed, through Christianity sharply separating itself from the earth, and defining spirituality in terms of the supernatural and unearthly. Because we distrusted our rootedness in the earth and its rhythms we learned to despise the body and sexuality. We can even speak of a cosmic matricide. And nowhere is this more evident than in Christian attitudes towards the ancient Mother Goddess. Now the last thing I want to do is to romanticise a supposed Golden Age of the Mother Goddess, when all was peace-loving, and men and women lived together in harmony. On the basis of a few statues in Anatolia and some cave-paintings we cannot re-create a culture. Especially when we have no written texts from this period. Nor is it the idea to suggest that matriarchy would be better than patriarchy or that we should reclaim for worship the deity of a lost culture. But we *can* look at the *matricentric* focus of some of these civilisations to understand what a Euro-centric Christianity has lost by rejecting an earth-centred culture. And my hope will be to restore the centrality of 'Care' to Christianity in a more holistic and transforming manner.

One of our first discoveries if we take the example of the Magna Mater Cybele, or Ceres, or Isis, worshipped in Greece or Ancient Rome, is that the link with *fertility* has always been rejected as 'pagan'. Secondly, the overpowering, irrational dimension associated with female sexuality associated with the worship of the Goddess has been distorted and demonised. This points to an underlying fear which Christianity can never quite overcome as to sexuality. We have needed to 'order' the world, through separating, through defining ourselves overagainst nature, body, emotion, feeling. All chaos, messiness, irrational spontaneity and disorder must be suppressed. Humanity, we are told, is *'capax Dei'*, but the divine element is reflected through the soul and not through the body. Hence it is no wonder that the Great Mother becomes the terrible Mother. And as such she has become a mythological, cross-cultural archetype. Both Jung and the neo-Jungian Edward Whitmont describe men's fear of the 'anima', the female personality type, embodied mostly by the mother:

> *"Fear and attraction, in fact, always go together in the confrontation of the world of the absolute other, the other sex... Even in the case of a good relationship between mother and son the pattern of expectation in regard to women has its element of secret fear."* [11]

This fear - verging on hatred - is best illustrated by another Jungian, Ernest Becker, in his book *'The Denial of Death'*. I cite it in full because I think this attitude underlies much of Christianity's rigid and stifling focus on motherhood:

> *"The real threat of the mother comes to be connected with her sheer physicalness. Her genitals are used as a convenient focus for the child's obsession with the problem of physicalness. If the mother is a goddess of light, she is also a witch of the dark. He sees her tie to the earth, her secret bodily processes that bind her to nature; the breast, with the mysterious sticky milk, the menstrual odours and blood, the almost continual immersion of the productive mother in her corporeality, and not least - something*

the child is very sensitive to - the often neurotic and helpless character of this immersion... The mother must exude determinism, and the child expresses his horror at his complete dependency on what is physically vulnerable. And so we understand not only the boy's preference for masculinity but also the girl's 'penis-envy'. Both boys and girls succumb to the desire to flee the sex represented by the mother; they need little coaxing to identify with the father and his world. He seems more neutral physically, more cleanly powerful, less immersed in body determinisms; he seems more 'symbolically free', represents the vast world outside the home, social world with its organized triumph over nature, the very escape from contingency that the child seeks."[12]

This passage sums up a hidden misogyny, the fear and loathing of female sexuality, the fear of embodiment, of dependency and vulnerability, and expresses the need to escape from nature and the world of the physical. Fear of the earthbound and decaying are projected onto the body of the mother. This matriphobia is also clearly seen in the anti-semitic cultural stereotyping of the Jewish mother.

On the other hand, Christianity spiritualised away the energies of the Great Mother. Jung himself realised how Christianity had transformed mother symbolism in the doctrine of the Assumption of Mary:

"The Christian Queen of Heaven has, obviously, shed all her Olympian qualities except for her brightness, goodness and eternality; and even her human body, the thing most prone to gross material corruption, has put on an ethereal incorruptibility... That being so, the question naturally arises... What has become of the characteristic relation of the mother image to the earth, darkness, the abysmal side of the bodily man with his animal passions and instinctual nature...?"[13]

What indeed? If we first recognize that the demonising of the Devouring Mother is a historical - not mythical - process of a way of coping with physicality and decay; and that conversely, the idealisation of one woman, Mary, as Queen of Heaven, does not touch the plight of real mothers, Christian theology can begin to de-mystify motherhood and allow richer meanings for caring to emerge. Once freed from the compulsion to define our Christian identity overagainst the rest of creation, more liberating models of caring - than that of motherhood based on self-sacrifice and suppression of more joyous sexuality, the female 'jouissance' - can spring into being.

3. Liberating new models of care

"a whole new poetry beginning here.
Visions begin to happen in such a life
as if a woman walked quietly away
from the argument and jargon in a room
and sitting down in the kitchen, began turning in her
lap
bits of yarn, calico and velvet scraps,
laying them out absently on the scrubbed boards
in the lamplight, with small rainbow-coloured
shells...
such a composition has nothing to do with eternity,
the striving for greatness, brilliance -
only with the musing of a mind
one with her body...
pulling the tenets of a life together
with no mere will to mastery,
only care for the many-lived, unending forms
in which she finds herself..."[14]

These words of the American poet Adrienne Rich evoke the notion of caring as a basic nurturing attitude towards all forms of life. Caring as tending, attending, as cherishing, as watching and paying attention to the 'many-lived, unending forms' and rhythms of ordinary living - rhythms of season and growth of myriad life forms; caring as commitment, as paying attention to the daily crucifixions of many peoples of the earth as well as the long-lived suffering of the whole of creation.

From this basic commitment springs an Ethic of Care, an Ethics of Responsibility, or as I prefer to call it, an Ethics of Connection. Ever since American educational psychologist Carol Gilligan wrote her book

'*In a Different Voice*', feminist thought has been developing an ethics of care and responsibility.[15] But Gilligan did not base such an ethic on an essentialist view of motherhood - although this has been the tendency of some influenced by her; rather on her research that the basis of moral decision-making of girls was different from that of boys. She developed her views in reaction to Lawrence Kohlberg, who saw ethics in terms of justice and fairness. On Kohlberg's scale girls appeared more confused and immature, boys more confident and 'mature' in their decisions. But Carol Gilligan showed that girls inevitably seemed more immature, *because they operated from a different basis, that of caring and responsibility*.

It is not my intention here to discuss the criticisms of Gilligan's theory; but I do want to draw attention, first, to the way she highlighted the gender distinction which operates at the basis of our moral decision-making. And, secondly, the way she used this to show that a different sense of self was also being developed. This I think is absolutely crucial for creating of new models of caring. For, far from being a rather middle-class, individualistic bourgeois notion of care, which has rightly been criticised for being limited to family, or one's immediate circle,[16] Gilligan showed that an ethic of care or responsibility is based on a more relational notion of the self, which I call "the connected self".[17] If I had time I could trace through myth and legend the way moral obligation and duty have been imaged in terms of detachment and separation. The hero is called by God to leave family, home, country, to a kind of heroic individualism and autonomy which is the opposite of attachment, depth of feeling, responsiveness, interdependence and qualitative interaction. And this is close to the model of caring I want to develop for Christian pastoral care. It is not a repetition of the old model of sticking to a contracted commitment, come what may: we have looked at some of the disastrous consequences of this.

Here is how a High School student described an ethic of responsibility: "Responsibility is when you are aware of others and aware of their feelings... Responsibility is taking charge of yourself by looking at others around you and seeing what they need ... and taking the initiative."[18] This student has a notion a self which grows through relationship, which defines itself empathically in terms of connection and relationship, instead of through distance, separation, control and detachment.

I see this as an enormous challenge: how can we re-define the developmental models by which we understand a child's growth to maturity - *with connection as their root metaphor rather than separation*? Can developing empathic skills and responsiveness in a variety of relationships - parent/sibling/friend/teacher - be the key to qualitatively different modes of caring which would never tolerate the marginalising and isolating of enormous numbers of wounded people? (I think here of the prison system, which is the ultimate form of isolation and wounding of a sense of self). From a Christian point of view, this is simply being true to the organic roots of Scripture - the vine and the branches, the members of the Body of Christ, the doctrine of the Trinity, and so on - in fact the lost mutuality-in-relating which I believe is the heart of the Gospel.

But, it will be objected, are you not falling into the very trap which you sketched to begin with? That women tend towards a relational notion of self and that this is our undoing? Two points need stressing: first, that the very skills of empathy, compassion and responsiveness in relation, need also to be practised on oneself.[19] And this is not easy. Especially when we have internalised the Christian ethic of self-denial, taking up the Cross and a concept of 'agape' which is detached and other-centred, the opposite of joyous eros. I think we have to understand that in all loving and compassion there is an element of 'self-interest' and pleasure - and this is indeed healthy. Mother-love is not and should not be totally other-centred: having a child, being in relationship, also meets a woman's needs and can be immensely satisfying. There are other modes of asceticism than in denying all bodily gratification! Society needs love, sacrifice, but not *self-sacrifice*: rather, we need structures of caring which cherish and nurture the self-in-relation.

Secondly, an ethics of connection does not focus solely on the interpersonal dimension - but on the communal and structural. Until our institutions - I think especially of health, educational and pastoral institutions, as well as the founding categories by which we understand human personhood - knowing, feeling, motivation and so on - show a willingness to transform the basis of their structures from controlling and ordering through detachment, objectivity and denial or trivialisation of connection, an ethic of connection as liberating model of care will make minimal impact.

And thus Woman-Church claims its open space.

From devouring mother to wounded healer

Our context is the safe space we make for each other where we acknowledge our brokenness; we see that we are wounded by the distorted stereotypes of being female, by the humiliation of female sexuality, by the over-focus on motherhood, and the interpretation of the mother as either a demonic earth-mother to be dismissed as pagan, the wicked step-mother who delivers the child to the wild beasts, or the angelic non-sexual virginal mother, who has lost contact with the earth and earthly desires. We have been broken by abusive family relationships, sometimes by those we most trusted, by wounds we have not dared to name.

But in our woundedness we are called to be healers. We are called to minister in mutuality to each other's brokenness. In our recovery of attending and tending to the lost rhythms and connectedness we are healers of each other. We re-discover 'care' through this recovery of connection. We are heard out of the depth into speech (the phrase is from the late Nelle Morton) by a listening of the heart, not by the speech of the expert. We minister to each other not through dependence on a distant hero-redeemer figure, or through dependent relationships which devour any possibility of sense of self, but through a kind of mutual messianism, where we participate in the relational, redeeming energy which was manifest in the life, death and resurrection of Jesus of Nazareth.

'Caring' is being present to each other in the pain of the particular memories. Think of the Dutch word 'herinneren', German 'erinnern', literally becoming present to the deepest parts of yourself. This is very

reminiscent of Augustine's 'Deus intimior intimo meo'! It is re-membering, interiorising our story. I mean, literally, in a culture and context
where dis-memberment is a cultural reality. Dismemberment in terms of
violence, in terms of being cut off from an empowering story of
origins - even our myths are dismembered. Our patterns of care have been
trivialised into the benevolence of a few individuals. 'Re-membering' is
literally putting new flesh on the bones, re-connecting with lost community memories, re-collecting, gathering up - you will notice that these
are all words with a strong ecclesial meaning - what has been lost, the
joyous, nurturing presence of God to creation in its entirety, the
humility, vulnerability and interdependency of being 'humus', 'homo',
adam, 'earthlings'.

If God is to be Emmanuel - truly at home in the Universe - then our
structures of caring in religion and society must embody our passionate
commitment to the interconnectedness of human well-being and ecological harmony.

References

1. Martin Heidegger, *Being and Time,* Oxford, Blackwell, 1962, tr. J. Macquar-
   rie and Edward Robinson, p.242.

2. See the foundational article of Elizabeth Schüssler-Fiorenza, Feminist
   Theology as a Critical Theology of Liberation, in Walter Burkhardt (ed),
   Woman: New Dimensions, New York, Paulist Press 1977, pp.19-50.

3. Rosemary Ruether, *Woman-Church - Theology and Practice*, San Francisco,
   Harper and Row, 1985, p.72.

4. Elizabeth Schüssler-Fiorenza, *Woman-Church: the Hermeneutical Center of
   Feminist Biblical Interpretation*. In: Bread not Stone, Boston, Beacon, 1984;
   Edinburgh, T & T. Clark, 1990, pp.1-22.

5. See Julia Kristeva, *Womens' Time*, in The Kristeva Reader, ed. Toril Moi,
   Oxford, Blackwell, 1986, tr. Alice Jardine and Harry Blake, pp.187-213; also
   About Chinese Women. In :ibid., tr. Sean Hand, pp.138-159.

6. Pope John Paul II, Apostolic Letter, *Mulieris Dignitatem*, Vatican City, 1984.

7. See Mary Grey, *Redeeming the Dream*, London, SPCK 1989; *Feminism, Redemption and Christian Tradition*, Mystic, Connecticut, 1990.

8. Pioneering work in this area is Jean Baker Miller's *Towards a New Psychology of Women*, Boston, Beacon, 1976; the work continues in discussions and papers produced by The Stone Center for Developmental Services and Studies, Wellesley College, USA - see Work in Progress Papers of Jean Baker Miller, Judith Jordan, Alexandra Kaplan, Janet Surrey etc.

9. I explored this in an article, *'Yet Woman Will be Saved Through Bearing Children: Motherhood and the Possibility of A Contemporary Discourse for Women'*. In: Bijdragen 52, 1991, pp.58-69.

10. The literature on the emerging of the Great Goddess in our times is enormous. A recent comprehensive study is Elinor W. Gadon, *The Once and Future Goddess,* Wellingborough, The Aquarian Press, 1990.

11. Edward Whitmont, *The Symbolic quest: Basic Concepts of Analytical Psychology.* Princeton, Princeton Univ. Press, 1969, p.192.

12. Ernest Becker, *The Denial of Death*, New York, Free Press, 1973, pp.39-40. I owe both these quotations to Demaris Wehr, *Jung and Feminism: Liberating Archetypes,* London, Routledge, 1988.

13. Cited by Demaris Wehr. In: *Ibid.*, p.112.

14. Adrienne Rich, *Transcendental Etude.* In: *The Dream of a Common Language,* New York, Norton and Norton, 1978, p.76.

15. Carol Gilligan. *In a Different Voice?* Harvard University Press, 1982; Nel Noddings, *Caring: A Feminine Approach to Ethics and Moral Education*, Berkeley and Los Angeles, Univ. of California Press, 1984. For critical discussion, see *Women and Moral Theory*, eds. Eva Kittay and Diana Meyers, New York, Rowman and Littlefield, 1987.

16. For example, by Susan Mendus, *Eve and the Poisoned Chalice,* unpublished lecture delivered at Nijmegen Congress of Womens' Studies, February 1991.

17. See Mary Grey, *Claiming Power-in-Relation: Exploring the Ethics of Connection.* In: Journal of Feminist Studies in Religion, Vol.7, no 1, Spring 1991, pp.7-18.

18. Cited in Carol Gilligan, *Remapping the Moral Domain: New Images of Self-in-Relationship*. In: Mapping the Moral Domain, eds. Gilligan et al, Harvard Univ. Press, 1988, p.7.

19. For the concept of self-empathy see Judith Jordan, *Empathy and Self Boundaries*, Stone Center Working Papers series, 1984.

Gospel and Pastoral Counselling in Africa

Wilhelmina J. Kalu

1. Introduction

Pastoral counselling in Africa is determined by the context or core facets of the environment: firstly, beyond the changing patterns of the formal level of culture characterised by education and skill acquisition, there is a persistence of the traditional world view. The philosophical and religious aspects of the culture determine a person's reaction when confronted with life's many surprises. Any viable model of counselling in this environment must take apt cognizance of this 'endurance of conviction'.

Secondly, from the earliest of Christian history in the Maghrib (Africa north of the Sahara) and from the Portuguese maritime enterprise in the 15th and 16th Centuries in Africa south of the Sahara, Christian forms from Europe sought to convert adherents of traditional African religions into a new model of explanation, prediction and control of space-time events. Varieties of interpretations of the Christian beliefs, ritual practices and ethical codes flooded the Continent. A host of strategies were employed. The score card showed that the introduction of the Bible in Africa made a revolutionary impact (AACC Report, 1978 and Mbiti, 1986). But Dickson and Ellingworth (1969) observed that

> *"It has become increasingly clear, and disturbingly so, that the Church has been speaking in Africa and to Africans in strange or partially understood tongues. We must be thankful to God that in spite of man's weaknesses and short-sightedness, the miracle of grace has been taking place all over Africa."* (Dickson and Ellingworth, 1969, p.9).

The short-sightedness referred to the negligence of the mental matrix of the African as well as to the deliberate, de-emphases of certain parts of the Bible, especially the pneumatological areas. The missionaries feared the problem of control in the move of the Holy Spirit and the spiritist character of the existing African religiosity. Indeed, Shorter (1975) endeavoured, in the wake of the Pope's declaration in Rubaga Cathedral, Kampala, Uganda, 1969, to seek for the path of dialogue between Christian and African spiritualities and for liturgical renewal. This is a reaction to a tidal wave of changes. The wind of change of the 1950's and 1960's which blew on the political plane created waves of cultural revivalism and posed the problem of indigenization in the churches. The cry was to make Christianity meaningful to the realities of the African environment.

Thirdly, contemporary religious scene in Africa is characterized by a) a successful entrenchment of indigenous non-white churches with a creative spirituality which the Africans have found attractive; b) a turbulence within the imported denominational churches which are suffering from low growth rate; c) a resurgence of evangelical Pentecostalism and charismatic movements which have endeavoured to redeem the failures of orthodox Christianity and to tap the pneumatological resources of the Bible. A re-evangelization of Africa is in progress. A good example is the 'Africa Must Be Saved' and Fire Convention which took place in Harare in 1985. This was organized by Evangelist Rheinard Bonkke. It brought together 4,000 preachers from 41 African countries in one tent which cost 800,000 dollars, for a massive training programme. This fanned the fire already spreading through Africa, (Gifford, 1986). As Peter Brierley (1991) has just demonstrated, the phenomenon is world-wide: orthodox churches are losing members while Pentecostals and charismatic churches are growing rapidly.

Fourthly, Africa has also been inflicted by a surge of eastern religions (Krishna, Guru-Maharaji, etc.), new science religions (Eckankar, Grail Message), theosophic clubs (Rosicrucian, AMORC) and the Lodges which hit the West Coast in the colonial period.

Amidst these religious forms, each proffering solutions to man's innumerable problems is a socio-economic and political backdrop which is turbulent. Civil Wars, political instability, huge external debts, famine and drought. All these have made life precarious in the African environment.

Admittedly, some have sought salvation in leftist ideologies, like communism, but most have sought the balm of Gilead in religious solace. Pastoral counselling in the African context must therefore take cognizance of this environment. The key question is the extent to which the gospel becomes a model and resource in effective pastoral counselling in this environment.

It must be quickly added that the gospel is not Christianity. The gospel is like the inside nut of the coconut. It is the life-giving nurture, the good news that Christ loves and saves. The salvation Christ offers is total. Christianity is like the shell of the coconut. It is a covering which is a process of presentation. It is therefore possible for culture to be a veritable vehicle as well as a hindrance. European cultural baggage often distorted the kerygma as Mbiti (1986) and Abogunrin (1988) demonstrated.

Some cultural forms can be against Christ, thus presenting the world with a 'christless' Christianity. This explains the New Testament warnings against the love of the world (Gk. cosmos) and the things in the world (Gk. kosmetikos). To do so is enmity with Christ. This is because the things of the world are embellishments, cosmetics with which the enemy of man dazzles, deceives and lure human beings into rebellion against God. Christ, therefore, judges all culture and reinforces the signals of transcendence in them for prospering the good news.

2. The African cosmology

The first task in African Pastoral Counselling is to reconstruct the world-view which influences the mental matrix of the African. Religious and material change-agents impact on this core sector. African cultures vary but a common denominator exists. *Space* is conceived as three-dimensional: the sky where the Creator and the major divinities (such as Thunder, Lightning, Sun and such-like) inhabit. These divinities are predominantly male and exude power. The Earth is under the ambit of the female Earth-Goddess. A number of spirits subserve as human spirits (for each person), patron spirits of various professions (hunting, agriculture, seafaring, etc.), nature spirits inhabiting matter, like trees, rocks, animal spirits in lions, tigers, rats, and evil spirits. Evil spirits are ubiquitous and could be tapped for the anti-social: witchcraft, sorcery, poisoning, infertility, mental illness. Particularly obnoxious is the child spirit which manifests as a child but is in fact sent to torment a woman only to return into the spirit world at a short-lived appointed time. Achebe (1986) studied the Igbo phenomenon of Ogbanje. The Yoruba call it *Abiku*. The Ga in Ghana call it *Gbobalō*.

Sharing the Earth is Water which is a world of its own replicating the Land. Mermaid spirits both male and female are known to operate under the Queen of the Coast. It is a female dominated sector. Mermaid spirits worship is widespread in Africa.

Beneath the Earth is the Land of the Spirits. Death is the door into this world. It is a dynamic existence and a mirror of the human world. Those who had lived good life on the earth and received proper burials, pass through it and reincarnate in due time with unspecified duration, into the human world for another life in a cyclical conception of time. Those who died bad deaths through suicide, small-pox, lightning and such inexplicable deaths, or lived wicked lives on earth, or were denied ritually acceptable burials, *cannot* reincarnate. They turn into evil, angry spirits poised to revenge on their progenitors on earth. This explains why certain sicknesses and misfortunes are explained by appeal to the anger of one's ancestors. Happy ancestors use their spiritual powers to protect and give good fortunes to their scions on earth. These, in turn, recipocrate by sharing food and drinks in libations and prayers with ancestral spirits (Gaba, 1973). Kilson has provided analyses of prayers and libations among the Ga, also of Ghana. Shorter (1975b) and Mbiti (1975) have also given fuller studies of prayers among the Africans. For the most part, this domain is male controlled. In terms of gender, both sexes are fully recognized and accorded importance in invocation and worship. But this world-view is a precarious vision of human existence as it perceives a world under siege by evil spirits. Human beings, oblate, propitiate and seek the powers of the beneficent gods to ward off the attacks of the evil powers, to enhance the battle of existence and to control space-time events. It is an alive universe. It recognizes the hidden warfare underneath the material, existentialist life.

Causality is explained by appeal to this hidden warfare instead of empirical analysis (Kalu, 1978).

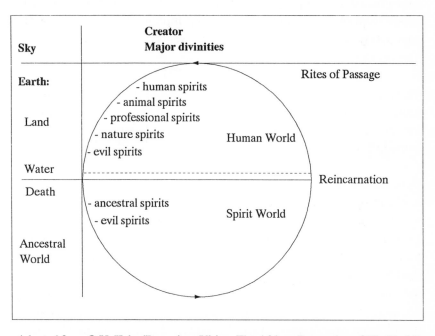

Adapted from O.U. Kalu, 'Precarious Vision: The African Perception of His World' in Kalu, *Readings in African Humanities: African Cultural Development* (Enugu: Fourth Dimensions Publishers Ltd., 1978).

In this seamless web of reality, there is no dichotomy between the sacred and profane. The enduring problem of the pastoral counsellor in Africa is how to bring the gospel imperatives as a resource to the needs of a person who holds on to the above-sketched world-view.

3. The New Testament world-view

A prelude would seek to ascertain whether there is a clash of world-views between the New Testament background of the gospel and the African context. There is an inner unity between the Old and New Testaments, the latter is a fulfilment of the former. The perception of time in the Old Testament is cyclical as in the African environment. Eliade argues that the cyclical pattern is borrowed from the agricultural cycle and is common to a predominantly agricultural level of human civilization. The New Testament salvation history is built on a linear perception of time, moving from the past through the present to a future aeon. However, in the incarnation of Christ, the not-yet-period intervened into the here-and-now period. Diagrammatically, it is represented as follows:

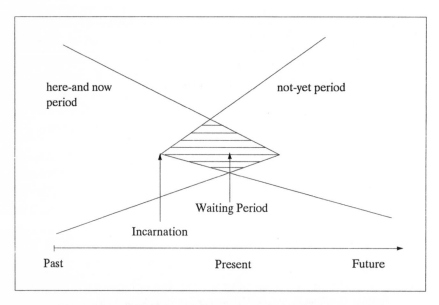

Adapted from O.U. Kalu, *Missionary Strategies in Africa in the 1980's*
(Geneva, Lutheran World Federation, 1980).

The Kingdom of God with enormous resources for liberation of mankind from the captivity of demonic forces has come into the midst of mankind. He is the Emmanuel, God with us, dwelling among men. He is the Jehova Shamma (Ezekiel 48:35) who is ever present. But the fullness shall yet appear when this aeon closes and the rapture occurs. The present is a dynamic one and is the scene of End Time battle.

Thus, in spite of the structural differences in the contrast between cyclical and linear time frames, time in New Testament is not abstract, it is *kairos* - time as event. This is similar to the African perception. Secondly, the New Testament avoids a dichotomy just as the African does. Rather, events in the existential reality is understood by operative forces in the spiritual realm. For one, God is a spirit and those who worship can only do so by operating in the spiritual realm. In that realm resides truth and the true life, Jesus. Paul put the matter rather tersely in Romans 8:5-9

> *"For they that are after the flesh do mind the things of the flesh; but they that are after the Spirit the things of the Spirit. For to be carnally minded is death; but to be spiritually minded is life and peace. Because the carnal mind is enmity against God: for it is not subject to the law of God, neither indeed can be. So then they that are in the flesh cannot please God. But ye are not in the flesh but in the Spirit, if so be that the Spirit of God dwell in you. Now if any man have not the Spirit of Christ, he is none of his."*

Paul moves to develop the doctrine of the two kingdoms: one is controlled by Satan and the other by Christ. There is no medial position for human beings. A person is in either one city or in the other. Salvation is a military term signifying the rescue operation or liberation of captives from Satan's kingdom into God's kingdom. Christ declared in his first sermon that this was his basic task or mission to the earth. God was in Christ reconciling a lost world unto Himself.

A second contention of Paul is similar to the African, namely that human life is a precarious existence as evil spirits or demonic forces seek to ruin the happiness of life. He encouraged the Ephesians to

> *"be strong in the Lord and in the power of his might. Put on the whole armour of God, that ye may be able to stand against the viles of the devil. For we wrestle not against flesh and blood, but against principalities, against powers, against the rulers of darkness of this world, against spiritual wickedness in high places."* (Eph. 6:10-12).

The implication is that Satan is organized in a hierarchy: some of his agents are *principalities* commanding a host of *powers*, who, in turn, control a plethora of rulers of darkness, other agents who perpetrate wickedness in high places and down to demons. In other passages, specific names and identities are provided, the cohort in the marine world are enumerated and details of their strategies are exposed to warn the Christian. Paul admonishes the Christian to be alert and ready as an athlete, an active farmer or a soldier under arms. An incautious, unprepared moment could prove devastating because the enemy goes around, like a roaring lion, seeking a victim to devour.

The New Testament world-view is intensely spiritual. Nothing happens in the physical world which has not been ordained either in the kingdom of darkness or in the kingdom of light where Christ rules, sitting on the throne with his holy angels around him (Matt. 25:31).

The ethical implication is obvious. Man cannot by his own ability confront the enemy. The strength of the Lord and the power of his might is the refuge. This means an ethical life pattern consonant with a close relationship with a holy God. The African Christian seeks to live a life free from filthiness of body and spirit (2 Cor. 7:1) just as the African non-Christian hedges himself with taboos and ritual purity so as to enable him tap the aid of beneficent Gods against evil spirits. The African Christian seeks Jesus as the provider, and the non-Christian sacrifices to spirits for wealth and titles. Explanation of causality is similar in both; ethical implications are identical. There are, however, significant, inner differences in spirituality: Does the African god love? Does the African love his gods? This is a major difference because African worship of deities is heavily materialistic. One brings a lot of offerings to his god to consult him. A threat can therefore be made in a prayer that if the god did not perform, the groves of the shrine would soon be overgrown. In the New Testament, God loves and gives and gives. He demands love as a pre-requisite to a healthy relationship. The love should flow to our fellow men because if one cannot love those whom one sees, how can one love God whom one does not see. This is both a relief to the African and fits into his communal caring life style.

It is evident that missionaries preferred the Bible as a source of under-standing God and yet proceeded to ignore some parts of it. As the Bible became more available in the African environment, eyes opened and the spiritual dimensions were now perceived as possible resources for meet-ing the challenges and needs of the African environment. The indigenous non-white churches were the first to perceive these potentials. But they allowed much of the uncleaned African forms to intrude. The Pentecos-tals are now removing the dross and tapping the biblical resources using *only the Bible* (sola scriptura). They are, therefore, growing.

Hollenweger (1972, 1980, 1986, 1990) has in a number of studies sought to explain the growth of the non-indigenous churches as well as the Pentecostals in the Third World. He pointed to certain characteristics which dovetailed to the Third World environment and elicited interest:

1. nonconceptual medium of theologizing - song, dance;
2. an alternative or a complement to western medicine - prayer for the sick. This is based on an understanding of body/mind relationship that is informed by experiences of correspondence between body and mind;
3. an exploration into the dark side of the soul - exorcism or deliverance;
4. a cathedral of sounds: glossalalia;
5. maximum participation at the levels of reflection, prayer, decision-making and, therefore, a form of community that is reconciliatory;
6. inclusion of dreams and vision into personal and public forms of worship - they function as a kind of icon for the individual and community.

Hollenweger does not fully appreciate the attack of the Pentecostals on the independent churches. Hastings (1989) in his study of Archbishop Milingo operates on the same unified hypothesis. He sees a close rela-tionship in idiom to Mutunwa Church of the healer, Peter Mulenga. Similarity in idiom should not obscure a core difference in spirituality. Pentecostals are aware of spirits which are not of God but rather fake (1 Jhn. 4:1-2; Is. 19:3). This is a disguise of Satan. Pentecostals argue in the African context that instruments such as holy water, candles, sacri-fices, oil and such like are cultic and syncretic. They insist that the power of the Word of God alone is enough to heal and save. These differences are important for pastoral counselling based on the gospel and operating in the African context.

4. Christian revival movements

A new awakening to the Bible has led to widespread evangelisation of Africa (AACC Report, 1978). This has led to renewal and revival movements within the denominational Churches in both East and West Africa (Rostedt, 1982). There are several reasons for these. The main ones include, firstly: the Bible is considered a deliberate choice in life-response within the African environment. Secondly, the "power of the Word of God"-approach offers a release from a host of moral and worship disorders that have invaded Christian Churches in Africa. Thirdly, the Apostolic, old time Christ-centred communal life is relevant to African communal life, where all are brethren and are to help each other to survive the physical and spiritual life race.

The need for continuous care and support of members or converts have helped in the establishment of Holy Spirit-power controlled ministries and neighbourhood fellowships.

There is emphasis on being born again spiritually, spiritual deliverance and power for Christian living through the infilling of the Holy Spirit and the Word of God (Rostedt, 1982). A notable aspect is that there is an attack on these groups from both within the Christian fold (The Western based churches) and those outside of it. Despite these the growth is significant (Hackett). These changes bring new dimensions to pastoral care and counselling in Africa. Since Pentecostal/revival movements constitute the cutting edge in contemporary African Christianity, it is pertinent to examine more closely the models of pastoral care and counselling which they employ. This is crucial because Cobb (1977) has shown the tendency of pastors in 'orthodox' or 'mainline' churches to appropriate on humanistic psychology in counselling models.

5. Models of Christian pastoral care in Africa

Life in Africa is communal and individual growth and self-realisation are largely expressed in the context of the community, that is the welfare of others (Kalu, 1989, 1991). The members of a community of faith in Africa are multi-ethnic and multi-lingual. They cut across racial, social, economic, educational and political characteristics. The numbers are necessarily large. Different models of pastoral care and counselling are therefore applied. A few models operate with paid workers and these are those involving parish and ordained ministers. The other models operate with non-paid workers, tent-makers or those earning salaries else-where. A dominant feature is the "workers in the vineyard" approach or "tending the flock". It fits into the idea of community in the Judeo-Christian tradition (Turner, 1987).

a. Parish Minister based Counselling

Most Africans take their religion seriously. Christians and non-Christians alike approach parish ministers to seek a Bible-based approach or God's solution to a plethora of problems. These include infertility, marital infidelity, chronic ill-health, bereavement, inability to marry. They often seek informed opinion on the host of avenues offered in the community for solving these problems, like the herbalist, prayer houses.

The untrained parish minister in pastoral counselling, mainly listens, comforts and prays for clients. The trained parish minister through a few courses in bible school or theological seminaries, may use other therapeutic approaches, known in the Western world. Family therapy is practised with a peace-making orientation rather than confrontational. It is also practised with the welfare of the group as a priority which is attained with cognisance to individual differences. Counselling by the parish minister takes place in his office, in the church premises, anywhere he is met in the community, and in visits to family homes. He is consulted in times of birth and death and for education on church procedures. He visits afflicted members in hospitals and schools. He therefore serves as a hospital or school chaplain as the occasion demands.

b. Elders Counselling

Church establishments tend to have elders (II Tim. 5:1, 17; James 5:14; Titus 1:1-9; II Pet. 5:1-3). They have members of the congregation assigned to them in zones. They visit, generally encourage, exhort and share the family concerns as they occur, as well as help to determine the response of the Church to a situation needing communal effort. Such include market-fire disasters for traders, feeding, clothing or paying school fees for children in a bereaved family. Elders keep in touch with members to provide preventive counselling. Interventive counselling is initiated by elders and taken over by parish ministers. Their qualification is experience in church matters, love of the flock of Jesus, and knowledge of the Word of God. They visit their clients or wards with delegations from the congregation when in hospitals and hometowns as the need arises.

Parish ministers, elders and congregational counsellors may make referrals to professional therapeutic counsellings, like doctors, psychologists, guidance counsellors.

c. Congregational Counselling

This is largely an ad hoc arrangement of counselling and care during crises periods, illness, death, robbery, birth, marriage rites. The composition of the group changes with each situation. The selection of the group changes with each situation. The selection may be made by church leaders or by individuals themselves if they consider sharing an intimate relationship with the member in need. Their strength is that they can stay and sleep with the person or family for days until he/she is able to cope on his own again. Their disadvantage is in supplying a host of well-meaning advice that may not be helpful. Congregational counselling is an effective task force in pastoral care and counselling in Africa. Membership of the flock is large and covers varieties of educational backgrounds, careers and life experiences. These are effectively tapped to the benefit of an individual in a faith community.

> *"Who also hath made us able ministers of the New Testament; not of the letter; but of the spirit ... the spirit giveth life."* (II Cor. 4:6)

d. Fellowship Counselling

This is usually counselling based on salvation, repentance, deliverance, message of Christ (Mk. 16:15-18). Afflictions are handled on a soul-spirit-body approach. A dominant feature of this approach is the empowerment of the Holy Spirit or the manifestation of ministerial gifts (Paton, 1960). There is prayer and deliverance supplemented by bible studies either on individual or group basis. This operates often in the place of fellowship, but sometimes in the home as well.

Problems of afflicted individuals are approached with the Word of God and prayers. Situations are anchored in relevant biblical passages in the Word of God which is eternal (Jhn. 8:51). There are monthly pro-grammes, crusades, weekly activities and some have 24-hour counselling service. The counsellors are often those with ministerial gifts (healing, helps, teachers). They come from a wide range of educational and career sources, like medical practitioners, University professors, teachers, scientists, professionals, business men, traders and artisans. The major qualification is the manifestation of the knowledge of the Word of God and the power of God through them. But they are controlled by a formation set up in the fellowship to monitor and approve such counsel-ling and care activities. Their term of office is therefore not indefinite.

Many of these neighbourhood ministries grow phenomenally into Minis-tries with a wide national and international coverage. They are within walking or travel distance in the community. They often practise the Apostolic life-style (Acts 4). A number of the clients are individuals who have faced unsatisfactory approach to their problems, therapeutically through Christians, psychological helps, spiritist, traditional divination and cult practices. Case histories are quickly turned into testimonies on goodness of God in complete healing, cure, deliverance and provision of needs. There are babies for the barren and those without womb, poor heart conditions made whole, eye-sight restored, cancer cured, as well as lame walk and deaf hear. Many of these receive medical confirmations as well. Spiritual afflictions and demonic attacks on whole families receive total deliverance whether from witchcraft, familiar and mermaid spirits (Isaacson, 1990).

Many ministries in Africa are headed by leaders from most unlikely sources like professors, scientists, medical doctors, professionals. They include W.F. Kumuyi (Mathematician) in Deeper Life, Pastor Adejare Adegboye (Professor of Mathematics) in Redeemed Christian Church in Nigeria, Zacharias Tanee Foomun (Professor of Organic Chemistry) in University of Yaounde, Cameroon, Ibeneme (Professor of Gynaecology) in Faith Clinics, Nigeria and Abani in Zaire. The current Church membership in such congregations varies from 200 to 8,000. Gatherings of 5,000 are common for worship purposes. Many have huge halls and auditoriums to accommodate members. Counselling services are also offered through radio teachings, newsletters, magazines and Sunday newspapers and devotional literature. Members or clients often join other fellowship groups within their own occupational/professional associations, lunch groups in offices for a network of continued growth and support.

e. Psychological Counselling

Psychological counselling occurs with practitioners trained in western therapeutic models. These may be psychologists and guidance counsellors in the Church membership, who are called upon or encouraged to offer counselling services in aid of individuals and families with problems. The bulk of such services are offered on volunteer basis. Few of these practitioners could be ordained ministers or those trained specifically in pastoral counselling and hospital chaplaincy.

Most of the services offered are on family and marital therapy. Ecclectic approaches or major therapeutic models including psychotherapy, behaviour modification and risk growth models may be used (Masamba and Kalu, 1989). These emphasis change, dependent largely on the individual.

There are also established Christian Family Counselling Ministries. These include Odunze's Family Circle (Odunze, 1989), Ijagbulu's Olu-Ibukun Foundation (Ijagbulu, 1985) in Nigeria, and the Christian Council of Ghana. Such establishments offer systematic seminars and workshops on all areas of family issues and concerns. There is a marriage between basic bible teachings and psychological principles guiding intra-family relationships. The topics of seminars include origin of marriage and family life, responsibilities of the woman, of the man, basics in keeping relationships going, basic problems of youth, marriage preparations, parent-child relationships. These services are highly sought for and these counsellors operate a heavy schedule of engagements with a lot of travelling involved. Their counselling materials are produced in books, tapes, magazines. The Olu-Ibukun Foundation has a strong outreach to youth in schools, up to the universities. They believe in operating in the helps ministry (II Cor. 12) and have at least four counselling departments, premarital, family, educational and vocational. Once more, sharing of testimonies (successful case-studies) and use of common questions asked by a target group of clientelle have proved effective in their counselling work (Ijagbulu, 1985).

These models suggest a problem: most of the practitioners do not have formal training in psychology and rely on revelation and the gifts of the Holy Spirit while professional counsellors insist on psychological theories. At issue is biblical anthropology (1 Thess. 5:23) which perceives the soul as warring against the spirit. Thus, Pentecostals seek the release of the spirit as a means of salvation and healing.

Some Common Problems in Christian Pastoral Care and Counselling

It is important to note that the fast growth rate in Church membership in Africa ensures that all the models co-exist and there are many more in development. The pastoral counsellor is careful not to disappoint in the spiritual search of the individual. Those who are dissatisfied move to the spiritist churches and traditional healers to participate in a host of sacrificial rituals and 'special' prayers.

The priest as a pastoral counsellor is often seen as a model to identify with. His own testimony is important for those who have to share life in similar situations. This creates shattering experiences when moral disorders, contrary to biblical teachings are observed in such models. Many priests in orthodox denominations do not have basic interest in pastoral counselling, and view with suspicion those who approach Church for financial help. They prefer duties that yield financial resources like baptism, funerals and marriages. Conferences on pastoral work dynamics are ill attended but those on marriage, baptism rites are well attended. In such cases, vehicles provided for ministers' use in pastoral care get used for personal purposes mainly. Such ministers practise "absentee visitation" which is asking about families from a member of the congregation.

Similarly, there are commercial minded organisers of counselling ministries based on the gospel or Word of God approach. Negative reactions of orthodox (un-renewed) mainline Churches to the wave of revivalism and Holy Spirit power spread have been unable to stem the tide or reduce the rate of growth in Pentecostalism. Several members of such congregations belong to fellowship ministries as well, a sort of dual or multiple-membership in Christian faith communities.

Conclusion

Africa has always been a spiritual terrain. The wind is blowing. There is a move from believing just in God and walking with him, to believing in Jesus and walking with him. There is a move from half-measure gospel to full-measure gospel, from gospel in script to gospel in power. There is therefore a move from powerlessness to transform the individual self in the face of plethora of spiritual and material problems to an era of dependence on the transforming power in the love of God, in Jesus. God and Jesus as the counsellor become a reality. The more intense and complex the problem is, the more the belief in divine intervention.

The communal life pattern in African tradition and belief in man as a spirit being are receptive to what the bible offers in the Old and New Testament teachings. The God of love of the bible is a relief from the demanding angry gods of ancestral Africa, that need to be appeased with every move of man. The gospel becomes an ever current good news that has dominion over circumstances and works of darkness. The main purpose of the Holy Spirit outpouring is to inaugurate an era in which men can call on the name of the Lord on their own and be saved (Joel 2).

"Therefore say I unto you. The kingdom of God shall be taken from you and given to a nation bringing forth the fruit thereof." (II Pet. 2:16 KJV)

References

AACC Report, *The Bible and the Evangelisation of Africa.* Limuru, Kenya, 1978.

Abogurin, Samuel O., *The First Letter of Paul to the Corinthians: African Bible Commentaries.* Ibadan, Daystar Press, 1988.

Achebe, Chinwe C., *The World of the Ogbanje.* Enugu, Fourth Dimension Publishers, 1986.

Brierley, Peter, *Christian England.* London, Marc Publication, 1991.

Cobb, John, *Theology and Pastoral Care.* Philadelphia; Fortress Press, 1977.

Dickson, Kwesi and Ellingworth, Paul (eds), *Biblical Revelation and African Beliefs*, Maryknoll, Orbis Books, 1969.

Gaba, Christian, *Scriptures of an African People: The sacred Utterances of the Anlo.* New York, NOK Publishers, 1973.

Gifford, Paul, Africa shall be saved. *Journal of Religion in Africa* 1987, 17, 63-92.

Hackett, RC., *New Religions Movements.*

Hastings, Adrian, *African Catholicism: Essays in Discovery.* London: SCM Press, Chapter 9, 1989.

Hollenwerger, W.J. , *The Pentecostals.* London, 1972.

Hollenwerger, W.J. , *Charismatic Renewal in the Third World: Implications for Mission.* Occasional Bulletin 1980, 4, 2, 68-74.

Hollenwerger, W.J., *After Twenty Years in Pentecostalism. International Review of Mission* 1986, 75, 297, 3-12.

Hollenwerger, W.J., The Theological Challenge of Indigenous Churches. In: A.F. Wallsand, W.R. Shenke (eds). *Exploring New Religions Movements: Essays in Honour of H.W. Turner Ekhart,* Indiana; Mission Focus 1990, 163-168.

Iljagbulu, Dele O., *Teenagers and Sex: Volume One.* Ibadan, Olu-Ibukun Publications, 1985

Isaacson, Alan, *Deeper Life: The extraordinary growth of the Deeper Life Church.* London, Hodder and Stoughton, 1990.

Kalu, Ogbu U. Precarious Vision: The African Perception of his World. In: O.U. Kalu (ed). *Readings in African Society: African Cultural Development* Enugu, Founa Dimension Publishers, 1978.

Kalu, O.U., *Missionary Strategies in Africa in the 1980's.* Geneva, Lutheran World Federation, 1980.

Kalu, W.J., Widowhood and its Process in contemporary African Society: A psycho social study. *Counselling Psychology Quarterly* 1989, 2, 2, 143-152.

Kalu, W.J., *Woman as an Individual in African Family Dynamics.* (Unpublished paper), 1991.

Masamba, Ma Mpolo and Kalu, W. (eds), *Risks of Growth: Pastoral Care and Counselling in African Context.* Nairobi, Kenya. Uzima Press, 1985.

Mbiti, J.S., *New Testament Eschatology in an African Background.* Oxford, Oxford University Press, 1971.

Mbiti, J.S. *The Prayers of African Religion.* London, SPCK, 1975.

Mbiti, J.S., *Bible and Theology in African Christianity.* Nairobi. Oxford University Press, 1986.

Odunze, Don, *Family Circles Seminars and Workshop Handbook.* Enugu, Family Circle Publication, 1989.

Paton, David M., *The Ministry of the Spirit: Selected Writings of Roland Allen,* 1968.

Rostedt, M., The Revival Movement in East Africa. *Africa Theological Journal* 1982, 2, 1, 63-84.

Shorter, Alyward. *African Christian Theology.* London, Geoffrey Chapman, 1975a.

Shorter, Alyward. *Prayer in the Religious Tradition of Africa.* Nairobi, Oxford University Press, 1975b.

Introduction Main Speakers

Dr. Jorge Cardenas Brito worked as psychiatrist and became minister in the Presbyterian Church of Chili in 1990.

Dr. Maarten den Dulk was Dean of the Theological Seminary of the Nederlandse Hervormde Kerk at Driebergen, The Netherlands. His church recently appointed him as professor of Practical Theology at the University of Leiden.

Dr. Edwin H. Friedman is an ordained Rabbi and a practising family therapist. He served as Rabbi of the Bethesda Jewish Congregation until 1979. He now conducts his own postgraduate training center for the clergy and other members of the helping professions in Bethesda, Maryland, USA.

Mrs. dr. Padmasani Gallup worked, until recently, in the Madras Diocese Church in India. She is now professor at the Madras Christian College and teaches Social Ethics.

Mrs.prof.dr. Mary Grey teaches at the Roman Catholic University of Nijmegen, The Netherlands. She has a chair in Feminism and Christianity.

Mrs.dr. Wilhelmina Kalu is Senior Lecturer at the University of Nigeria and Vice-President of the African Association on Pastoral Care and Counselling. She was trained as a family and child therapist.

DATE DUE

1/14/11			